Sleep Like a Baby

The Ultimate Guide to Better Sleep with Natural Remedies and Sleep Hacks

DR ADAM WELL

Copyright © 2023 Dr Adam Well
All rights reserved
No portion of this book may be reproduced in any form without written permission from the publisher or author, except as permitted by U.S. copyright law.

This publication is designed to provide accurate and authoritative information regarding the subject matter covered. The information presented in this book is intended for educational purposes only and does not constitute medical advice. While the publisher and author have used their best efforts in preparing this book, they make no representations or warranties with respect to the accuracy or completeness of the contents of this book and specifically disclaim any implied warranties of merchantability or fitness for a particular purpose. No warranty may be created or extended by sales representatives or written sales materials. The advice and strategies contained herein may not be suitable for your situation. You should consult with a professional when appropriate. The information presented is not intended to replace professional medical advice and treatment. Always consult with your health care physician before making any changes to your current treatment plan and before starting any new supplements, remedies or treatment even if it's a natural or herbal remedy, and before starting any new diet or health programs. Neither the publisher nor the author shall be liable for any adverse effects or consequences or loss of profit or any other commercial damages, resulting from the use of any suggestions or procedures discussed in this book.

Download your free companion guide including a sleep log and find additional resources at HealthMasteryLab.com/Sleep

Dedicated to my loving family whose love and support have been one of the greatest blessings in my life. To my mother who would always remind as a young child to be grateful for what I have as she tucked me in at night. And to all of us who have at one point struggled to get a good night's rest. I hope this book will serve as a helpful guide for you to achieve the restful sleep you deserve.

Table of Contents

1. Introduction: The Importance of Sleep................................1
2. The Problem of Insomnia 5
3. Sleep Hygiene 17
    Creating a Sleep Conductive Environment...............19
    Establishing a Regular Sleep Routine..........................21
4. Exercise, Diet, and Sleep 24
5. Stress, Meditation, Yoga and Stretching........................37
    Mindful Meditation..39
    Progressive Muscle Relaxation....................................42
    Yoga 43
    Stretching..44
6. Technology and Sleep 51
7. Natural Remedies for sleep 61
8. Aromatherapy and Sleep..70
9. Homeopathic Remedies for Sleep 87
10. Supplements for Sleep..93
11. Sleep Hacks for Better Sleep..104
    Autogenic Training..105
    Guided imagery 107
    Breathing Exercises..108
    Visualization Techniques 112
    Sleep-Inducing Foods and Drinks............................114
    Tools for Better Sleep...116
    Getting Lots of Sunshine During the Day..............123
12. Other Notes & Special Considerations 126

Napping 127
Managing Jet Lag 129
Night Shift and Sleep 132
Sleep Diaries 136
13. Conclusion 139

Chapter 1

Introduction: The Importance of Sleep

Similar to food and water, sleep is an essential human requirement. It is vital for our physical, mental, and emotional health. Sleeping well is important for maintaining optimum health and performing at our best during the day. Research have shown that adequate sleep of high quality reduces stress, promotes alertness, boosts immunity, and improves cognitive performance. Yet, sleep deprivation is a common problem, with many struggling to get enough sleep during the night. Even for those who do get enough hours of sleep, the quality may still be an issue. This lack of quality of sleep has a multitude of consequences on our health.

In addition to helping us feel rested and revitalized, sleep delivers various health benefits. While we're sleeping, our bodies conduct numerous processes that are vital to our health and well-being. Here are some physical and mental advantages of good healthy sleep:

Enhances Brain Performance

Improved brain function is one of the most significant benefits of adequate sleep. Sleep facilitates the consolidation of memories, the processing of information, and the development of new neural connections. Therefore it plays a major role in enhancing cognitive function, decision-making abilities, and creativity.

Improves Mood and Psychological Wellness

Improved mood and mental health are additional key benefits of quality sleep. Sleep deprivation has been associated with depression, anxiety, and other mood problems. Enough sleep can assist regulate emotions and lessen the symptoms of various mental disorders. It is fairly common for individuals who receive treatment for their insomnia to see a considerable reduction in depressive and anxious symptoms.

Aids in Cellular Healing and Rejuvenation

Moreover, sleep of quality is vital for physical performance. Your body repairs and regenerates tissue, produces hormones, and conserves energy while you sleep. This procedure is essential for maintaining a healthy immune system and sustaining normal body function.

Decreased Chronic Disease Risk

Also, research has demonstrated that high-quality sleep reduces the incidence of chronic diseases including obesity and diabetes. Insomnia has also been associated to an increased risk of cardiovascular disease, stroke, and hypertension. Adequate sleep reduces inflammation and stress in the body, which can enhance general health overall.

Helps Control Weight

Sleep plays a crucial function in regulating hormones that affect hunger and appetite, hence aiding in weight management. When we don't get enough sleep, our systems create more of the appetite-stimulating hormone ghrelin and less of the appetite-suppressing hormone leptin. This can eventually lead to overeating and weight gain.

Increases Energy and Productivity

A good night's sleep is necessary for sustaining energy levels and productivity during the day. When we are well-rested, we are more alert, able to concentrate better, and more capable of completing activities efficiently.

The optimal amount of sleep per day will vary from individual to another, and from one situation to another. That being said, most experts generally recommend 7-9 hours per day for most adults. Variables such as a person's genetic predisposition, the quality of their sleep, their lifestyle, and their overall health will determine how much more or less this person may require. It is crucial to consider how you feel throughout the day and how it relates to your sleep habits in order to assess if you are getting sufficient quality sleep. Without adequate rest, our bodies cannot function properly; we become sluggish and fatigued throughout the day due to a lack of energy, we are more likely to make errors due to impaired judgment and decision-making skills, we become emotionally vulnerable with an increased likelihood of feeling angry or frustrated, and our physical health may suffer from weakened immune systems, resulting in an increased risk for illness and injury.

There are several elements that might affect our capacity to get high-quality sleep; some are external, such as noise level or bedroom surroundings, while others are more internal, such as daily habits and lifestyle choices. This book is intended to serve as a guide to help you regulate these elements and use them to your advantage so that you can sleep well every night and wake up feeling energized and ready for the day!

Chapter 2

The Problem of Insomnia

Do you frequently experience difficulty falling or staying asleep, or experience daytime fatigue, irritability, and problems concentrating? If you responded affirmatively to this question, you may be one of the millions of people who suffer with insomnia.

Insomnia is a sleep condition that impairs an individual's ability to fall asleep and remain asleep. It is characterized by difficulties going to sleep, numerous awakenings during the night, and early morning awakenings without enough rest. Insomnia can be acute, with a short duration of a few weeks to a couple of months, or chronic, with a duration that lasts several months or longer.

Insomnia is a prevalent issue, affecting approximately 30% of the global population. It is believed that 10-15% of adults in the United

States suffer from chronic insomnia, while up to 30% experience periodic insomnia. Insomnia can affect individuals of all ages and genders but is more prevalent in women than men. Insomnia is also more prevalent in older adults due to changes in sleep patterns related to aging. Insomnia can have serious effects, causing daytime weariness, concentration difficulties, irritability, and mood disorders. Moreover, insomnia can impede work performance, social interaction, and life quality. People with chronic insomnia are also more likely to suffer from certain health issues and develop problems like heart disease, stroke, obesity, depression, and anxiety.

There are many causes, varieties, and other factors associated with insomnia. Having a better understanding of this common health problem will assist you in taking efforts to help fight it and improve your sleep and general health.

Reasons for Insomnia

A multitude of medical, psychological, and environmental variables can contribute to insomnia. Knowing the nature of these factors can be helpful in properly managing and treating insomnia. Consider the following categories:

Psychological Factors:

Psychological factors such as stress, anxiety, depression, and other mental health conditions can contribute to sleeplessness.

These elements might keep the mind active and impede relaxation, making it challenging to fall asleep. For example, a person who is anxious about job or family matters may find it difficult to relax and fall asleep.

Medical Conditions:

Several medical problems can cause insomnia. Obstructive Sleep Apnea, for example, and some other medical conditions will directly impede a person's ability to sleep. Usually, obstructive sleep apnea is accompanied with loud snoring, pauses in breathing during the night, and unexpected awakenings accompanied by choking. Other conditions, like chronic pain, gastroesophageal reflux disease, asthma and other respiratory illnesses, can one way or another negatively affects a person's sleep. With the discomfort and distress associated with these illnesses, it can be difficult to fall or stay asleep.

Medications:

Some drugs might disrupt sleep and lead to insomnia. Certain drugs used to treat high blood pressure, asthma, and depression are examples of that category.

Lifestyle Habits:

Bad sleep habits, such as irregular sleep schedules, excessive caffeine consumption, and lack of exercise, can also lead to insomnia. For example, drinking a lot of coffee shortly before bed might makes it difficult for many people to fall asleep.

Environmental Factors:

Environmental elements, such as noise, temperature, and light, can also disrupt sleep and lead to insomnia. A noisy bedroom or a room that is too hot or too cold, for instance, can make it difficult to fall asleep.

Types of Insomnia

Insomnia can be categorized in a variety of ways, however the following are some of the most prevalent ones:

Chronic vs. Acute Insomnia:

Duration is one of the criteria often used to classify insomnia. If it's a short-term problem, lasting less than three months, it's usually classified as acute insomnia. If the insomnia is for more than the three months, then it's considered chronic insomnia. Short term stress, worry, or situational circumstances, such as jet lag or a change in work schedule, are frequently associated with acute insomnia. Chronic insomnia, on the other hand, may have a more complex collection of underlying reasons, such as chronic stress, lifestyle habits, continuously uncomfortable environment, and sometimes medical issues and pharmaceutical use. Insomnia with a duration of less than one month is sometimes referred to as transient insomnia.

Onset versus Maintenance Insomnia:

Onset insomnia refers to trouble falling asleep at the beginning of the night. Many variables, including stress, anxiety, and a hyperactive mind, might induce this. Individuals with onset insomnia may feel wide awake even when they are physically exhausted. This might result in irritation and a feeling of helplessness, which can exacerbate the issue.

In contrast, maintenance insomnia refers to problems remaining asleep throughout the night. Individuals with maintenance insomnia may have frequent nighttime awakenings, difficulty getting back to sleep, and early morning awakenings. Many variables, including sleep apnea, medical illnesses, and drugs, might cause this. In some circumstances, people with maintenance insomnia may not be aware that they are awakening during the night, as these awakenings may be brief and may not significantly disrupt sleep.

Although these are the most prevalent types of insomnia, it is good to recognize that there are other, less common varieties as well. Some individuals, for instance, endure 'early morning awakenings insomnia' causing them to awaken feeling unrefreshed and exhausted. Individuals may also experience a combination of both difficulty falling asleep (onset insomnia) and multiple nighttime awakenings (maintenance insomnia).

Knowing the various types of insomnia may be beneficial as you follow through with the book and set up a plan for yourself. Fortunately, many of the treatments and sleep hacks we'll discuss in this book are effective for acute and chronic insomnia, as well as for onset, maintenance, and early morning awakenings insomnia.

Impact of Insomnia

Since sleep is so important, a lack of sleep is going to have negative effects on both our mental and our physical health. The negative effects of bad sleep can impact our work, relationships, and personal life on the daily. Some of its negative effects include:

Increased Risk of Depression and Anxiety:

A well known danger of insomnia is the increased risk of depression and anxiety that can be associated with it. According to studies, people with insomnia are more prone to develop certain mental health disorders than those who obtain their needed sleep. In fact, some studies show that treating insomnia can significantly reduce depressive and anxious symptoms.

Obesity and Other Chronic Health Conditions:

Another danger of insomnia is the increased risk of obesity and other chronic medical diseases, such as diabetes, cardiovascular disease and stroke risk. Because sleep is so important for regulating our hormones, insomnia can mean certain hormonal imbalances which can in turn lead to increased appetite and increased difficulty in maintaining a controlled blood sugar level.

Impaired Cognitive Functioning:

Lack of sleep can also impair cognitive performance. Some of these symptoms can appear relatively quickly after a few nights of sleep deprivation. Without adequate quality sleep, one may face problems with concentrations, memory, and reaction time. Some research even shows some correlation with chronic insomnia and dementia. Unfortunately, as the dementia gets worse, many times, the insomnia can get worse as well.

Negative Impact on Relationships and Work:

The negative effects of insomnia can extend beyond what our own health and affect our relationships and life at work. With chronic sleep deprivation, we tend to become more prone to anger, mood swings, irritability and other states that can negatively affect our relationship to people around us. Additionally, it can have a negative effect on our work performance and lead to lower overall productivity.

If you've ever had even just a few consecutive nights without good sleep, you've probably experienced some of these negative effects. You likely won't be feeling or acting at your best if you haven't had a good night sleep in a few nights, and usually you and those around you would be able to tell the difference in the way you act and conduct your life.

Diagnosing Insomnia

Getting an official diagnosis of insomnia typically requires a thorough review of your sleep patterns, medical history, and lifestyle habits. Your healthcare physician may request that you keep a sleep diary, or a journal in which you note the times you go to bed, wake up, and other factors, to help identify patterns and problems in your sleep.

In some cases, your healthcare provider may recommend a sleep study, or a polysomnogram, be done to confirm the diagnosis. In a sleep study, you'll basically go to sleep with a number of electrodes attached to your body, which function to monitor certain parameters as you sleep, such as your brain wave activity, heart rate, and other measurements. This can help in diagnosing insomnia and also in identifying certain underlying medical issues that may be contributing to it. In addition to the sleep study, your healthcare provider will probably inquire about any medications you're taking or other medical issues that could be contributing to your sleep difficulties. A physical examination or blood tests to rule out other underlying medical issues may also be done depending on your individual symptoms and medical history. If the insomnia is actually caused by another medical issue or a treatable underlying problem, then the appropriate treatment may start by treating the underlying condition that is causing in the first place. If there are no other identifiable medical issues, then there are still treatment options that target your ability to sleep and the insomnia itself.

Treating Insomnia

There are numerous therapy options available for insomnia. Alterations to one's lifestyle may be all that is needed for some, but for others medical treatment may be required. As always, consult with a physician before starting a new treatment regimen. Possible therapeutic options include:

Prescription Medications:

Prescription drugs are an option for insomnia treatment in the right candidate. Commonly used medications include benzodiazepines and other hypnotics. However, these drugs may cause negative side effects such as daytime sleepiness and dependency.

Alternative Therapies:

Alternative therapies, including acupuncture and cognitive-behavioral therapy (CBT), can be an option for certain patients with insomnia. CBT is a branch of psychotherapy that aims to look at how beliefs and thoughts affect behavior and can be an effective treatment for some people.

Lifestyle Modifications:

For many people, lifestyle modifications should be the cornerstone of their treatment. Lifestyle modifications are the main subject of this book, along with natural remedies and other sleep hacks and tools. Treating insomnia with lifestyle modifications has many advantages including:

    1) Little to no side effects: As we've mentioned above, one of the main issues with prescription drugs is that they can be associated with a number of negative side effects. On the other hand, with lifestyle modifications, one does not have to worry as much about these drug-associated effects.

    2) Long-term benefits: Lifestyle modifications, when done right, are usually going to have benefits that extend beyond the quality of your sleep and that extend into other areas of your health and wellbeing. Since bad habits and unhealthy lifestyle choices can play a key role in causing insomnia, changing and improving these habits and making better choices can address these causes at the root the problem resulting in long term benefits. Because these habits are fixed, the likelihood of developing future episodes of insomnia goes down as well.

    3) Cost effective and readily available: Certain changes are going to be easier than others, but regardless, those lifestyle modifications for the most part are going to be affordable and available for anyone who wants to give them try.

4) Greater control: With lifestyle modifications, you'll be in the driver's seat. You're the one who is making the change, and you can see what's working and what's not, so you're more in control. There is tremendous satisfaction and reward in knowing that you were able to improve your life by changing your habits and making different choices. With certain medications, some people will feel less in control, and can get a sense of dependency on the drug.

For many people, lifestyle modifications will be all they need to treat their insomnia. For others, lifestyle modifications on their own are not enough. For some adding certain natural remedies like aromatherapy, herbal teas, or certain supplements will do the trick, and still for others therapies such as prescription medications may be needed. Each case and each individual is a little different. However, even if a person does require medications or medical treatments, it is still beneficial to be aware of lifestyle modifications that can be used in conjunction with other treatments to address sleep issues. This is almost always better than relying solely on medications while ignoring other things that one can do to optimize their sleep pattern.

As we have seen in this chapter, insomnia can have a considerable impact on one's physical and mental health; therefore, it is crucial to treat it well. There are multiple forms and multiple causes of insomnia, but fortunately, we have multiple treatment options available as well. We'll discuss some of these options in the remainder of this book. We'll discuss some lifestyle modifications, natural therapies and we'll talk about a few sleep hacks for quick results. As a disclaimer, nothing in this book is meant to replace professional medical advice. You should always consult with your physician first before making any changes to your treatment plan.

Chapter 3

Sleep Hygiene

Whenever I consult a person about their sleeping habits, one of the first things I want to look at is their sleep hygiene. Sleep hygiene refers to basically their usual set of practices and habits before going to bed. What time do they go to bed? What are they doing before to prepare? What is their sleeping environment look like? Two of the most important aspects of good sleep hygiene are a welcoming and a peaceful sleep environment and a consistent sleep schedule. I know from personal experience, that going to bed at the same time each night can be difficult. Sometimes things pop up, family commitments, work obligations, and/or a new TV show on Netflix. I have heard many people say that they tried but simply just weren't able to stick to it. Even if you can't establish a consistent sleeping schedule, all is not lost, and there is a lot of other things and tools you can use to help you get the sleep you need. That being said, however, I would be amiss not to mention the value of adhering to a consistent sleeping schedule, given how beneficial this practice can be to those who do it. The good news, for those who find it really difficult, is that as people start implementing some of the other tools and tactics that we'll cover in this book, it's not uncommon for them to automatically find themselves developing a more regular sleeping schedule. Still, if you're not one of those people, you need not fret; there are plenty of other things you can do. The reason I wrote this book to contain a large of variety of tools and techniques, is because I know not everyone will resonate with each method. The idea isn't to take everything you read here and implement every single thing perfectly! Wouldn't that be nice!! But, the hope is, by going through the ideas presented here, you'll able to pick up a few practices that you can use to help take your sleep to the next level. In the end, it's not just about knowing what to do, it's about doing it, therefore as a reader, you should determine which strategy you believe will succeed and can envision yourself adopting. Some may be simple and quick, while others will require more preparation. These first two subjects covered in this chapter may require a bit more preparation, but they can be very beneficial when applied:

SLEEP LIKE A BABY

Creating a Sleep Conductive Environment

Your bedroom (or sleeping area) is your haven for a restful night's sleep. Creating a comfortable resting environment is a vital part of proper sleep hygiene. Establishing a conducive sleeping environment can help you fall asleep quicker, stay asleep longer, and awaken feeling refreshed. Here are some suggestions for creating an environment suitable to sleep:

1: Keep Your Bedroom Cool

The right temperature is important for obtaining a restful night's sleep. A chilly bedroom can help you fall asleep more quickly and remain asleep longer. For optimum sleep, try to adjust the temperature between 60 and 67 degrees Fahrenheit (15.5 and 19.4 degrees Celsius). If this is too cold for you, you might begin by decreasing the temperature slightly. For children and older adults a temperature of 66-70 degrees Fahrenheit (18.9 to 21.1 degrees Celsius) may be more ideal. I use blankets to keep myself warm. A ceiling fan can also be used to keep the room cool and circulate the air. Investing in bedding and pajamas that are breathable and moisture-wicking can also assist control your body temperature.

2: Make your Bedroom Dark

Light can disturb sleep by interfering with the body's natural sleep-wake cycle. Use blackout curtains or shades to prevent all outside light sources, including streetlights and the sunrise. Try a sleep mask if you are unable to completely darken your room. Remove all light-emitting electronic gadgets, such as smartphones and alarm clocks with bright displays.

3: Invest in a Comfortable Mattress and Pillows

Your mattress and pillows should support your body and aid in maintaining a healthy sleeping position. Change your mattress every seven to ten years, and your pillows every one to two years, or whenever they lose their form and hardness.

4: Remove Clutter from the Bedroom

A cluttered bedroom can make it tough to unwind and relax. Ensure that your bedroom is devoid of clutter and has only objects that encourage relaxation, such as a nice book, soothing music, or aromatherapy diffuser.

5: Choose the Right Bedding

Select bedding that is comfy, breathable, and appropriate to your own preferences. Try purchasing sheets, blankets, and duvets made from natural fabrics such as cotton or bamboo.

6: Minimize Distractions

Your bedroom should be a sanctuary for sleep, so eliminate any distractions that could keep you awake. This may involve technological items such as televisions and smartphones, as well as a noisy pet.

You may also opt to implement some of the additional strategies for enhancing sleep that we shall discuss in the future. For instance, we will discuss the use of a white noise machine, which can assist conceal outside sounds and create a calming environment. As we discuss these in the next chapters, you can decide which elements you'd like to incorporate into your bedroom.

Establishing a Regular Sleep Routine

Keeping a consistent sleep schedule can be quite beneficial for ensuring a restful night's sleep. It entails sleeping and rising at the same time every day, even on weekends. While this can be a difficult task for some people, most will find the result to be worth the effort. Like with everything else, you don't have to be 100% perfect to reap the benefits, but generally speaking, the more consistent you can be, the better. I try to go to bed around the same time each night. To me, this means attempting to go to sleep between 10 p.m. and 11 p.m.; however I occasionally stay up much later due to a prior commitment, travel, a business function, or a tv binge; sometimes until 2 or 3 in the morning. As long as I return to my regular schedule the next day, then this occasional deviation does not bother me much. Nevertheless, if I were to do this twice or three times per week, then I will definitely notice the difference.

One of the primary benefits of maintaining a consistent sleep pattern is that it helps regulate the circadian rhythm or internal clock of the body. The circadian rhythm is a natural mechanism that controls your sleep-wake cycle and helps regulates other biological processes, including hormone secretion, digestion, and metabolism. When you go to be bed and wake up at the same time each day, you're allowing your body to follow a predictable pattern and keep your circadian rhythm in sync. This will assist you in falling asleep more quickly and staying asleep longer, allowing you to wake up feeling refreshed and revitalized. Moreover, a regular sleep pattern can provide various other benefits. For instance, it can aid in appetite management, mood and performance enhancement and overall productivity.

Unfortunately, many individuals struggle to keep a normal sleep routine. Work and family demands can be unpredictable and prevent us from a adhering to an exact schedules. Even without those factors, some may have difficulty going asleep at a regular hour, especially if they have hectic or irregular schedule during the day. Yet, if you decide to make it a priority, there are ways to make the process easier. One strategy is to progressively change your bedtime and waketime in small increments over the period of several days or weeks until you get to your goal schedule. This will help your body adjust gradually to the new schedule. In addition, establishing a relaxing nighttime routine that includes things like reading, taking a warm bath, and practicing relaxation techniques can help signal to the body that it is time to wind down and prepare for sleep.

Those two methods alone, creating a comfortable sleeping environment and a consistent sleep schedule, can make a huge difference for most people. However, they might not be enough for everybody. Luckily, they don't have to be. There are plenty of other tools that we're going to talk about in the coming chapters. We'll continue by addressing some other lifestyle choices and modifications and talk about diet, exercise, stress and how they can affect your sleep. We'll talk about things one should do and things one should avoid before going to sleep. We'll then move on to natural remedies one can use including specific herbs, essential oils, or supplements that can be of benefit, and then we'll discuss other tools, quick hacks, and methods that can help you get better sleep. We'll then talk briefly about napping, jet lag and shift work and then in the conclusion we'll address how to put everything together and come up with a plan.

Chapter 4

Exercise, Diet, and Sleep

Mostly everyone knows that exercise can be great for our mental and physical health. The benefits of regular exercise are many; and include reduced risk of chronic diseases (such as diabetes, hypertension, and cardiovascular disease), better endurance, increased energy, and better weight management. Additionally, exercise can have a range of mental health benefits boosting mood, enhancing self-esteem and cognitive function, and improving signs of depression. Did you know however, that exercise can also improve your sleep? Studies have shown that regular exercise shorten the time it takes one to fall asleep while improving sleep quality, decreasing nighttime awakenings and increasing the quantity of deep sleep you get through the night! The circadian rhythm, that internal clock that regulates your sleep-wake cycle, is also influenced by exercise. Studies have showed that those who engage in regular exercise get better sleep than those who are less active.

Recommended Exercises for Better Sleep

When it comes to healthier sleep, not all forms of exercise are created equal. While any physical activity is usually preferable to none, some forms of exercise are more helpful than others for enhancing sleep quality. Running, walking, jogging, swimming, and other forms of aerobic exercise that increases the amount of oxygen delivered to your blood can help people fall asleep more quickly. Resistance training, such as weightlifting or utilizing resistance bands, helps increase the quality of deep sleep. Yoga, which combines physical poses with breathing exercises and meditation, can help you relax and reduce stress, which can enhance your overall sleep quality.

Exercise Timing for Better Bleep

It's not just about exercising, but getting the time right is also helpful. While there is no universally accepted truth to the topic of 'when to exercise' for best sleep, experts typically advise avoiding high-intensity exercise too close to bedtime. Vigorous exercise can raise your body's temperature, making it more difficult to fall asleep soon after. Several forms of exercises can increase the body's production of adrenaline and other stimulating hormones, which might disrupt the sleep-wake cycle if done too close to bedtime. For most people, high intensity exercise should be scheduled at least three hours before bedtime. Some individuals may find that exercising earlier in the day or in the morning is optimal. Nonetheless, gentle exercises like light yoga can help you unwind and relax in the evening, and you may find them beneficial even if performed closer to your bedtime.

The key here is to pay attention to your body and develop a training regimen that works for you. If you are not a morning person, it may not be sustainable to force yourself to work out early in the morning every day. Instead, try with various workout schedules to determine which is optimal for your body and sleep.

Regular exercise can be a potent technique for enhancing sleep quality. Exercise can help you fall asleep faster, remain asleep longer, and enjoy deeper sleep. Aerobic activity, resistance training, and yoga are all beneficial for improving sleep quality. It is crucial to select a fitness program that works for you because the timing and intensity of exercise might alter sleep quality. By incorporating regular physical exercise in the day, you can improve your health and your sleep quality at night

A Diet for Better Sleep

Just like exercise and physical activity, diet and nutrition can also have a substantial effect on sleep quality. Several individuals are unaware that what they eat and when they eat it might alter their ability to fall asleep and their quality of sleep during the night. In reality, certain foods and beverages can encourage relaxation and help the body prepare for sleep, while others might disrupt the sleep cycle and make it harder to fall asleep or remain asleep. In this part, we'll look at some of the better foods to consume for improved sleep.

Melatonin rich Foods:

Melatonin is one of the main hormones that our body use to help regulate and influence our sleep. It plays an important role in regulating our bodies' circadian rhythm, and eating melatonin-rich foods before bedtime can help suggest to our body that it's time to wind down. Melatonin-rich foods include tart cherries, walnuts, almonds, bananas, and kiwis.

High-Tryptophan Foods

Tryptophan is an amino acid that functions as precursor to serotonin, an important mood and sleep-regulating neurotransmitter. Eating foods rich in tryptophan can facilitate relaxation and enhance sleep quality. Turkey, chicken, eggs, cheese, nuts, and seeds are examples of tryptophan rich foods.

Magnesium-Rich Foods

Magnesium is an essential mineral for the body's ability to relax and fall asleep. Magnesium-rich food can help reduce stress and anxiety, allowing you to fall asleep faster. These foods include dark leafy greens like kale, spinach and collard, nuts, seeds, whole grains, and legumes.

Herbal Teas

Herbal teas have been used for centuries to help promote sleep and relaxation. We'll discuss those more in the coming chapters and talk about specific ones you might want to try.

Warm Milk:

Warm milk is a classic drink that has also been used for ages to help promote sleep. Milk contains tryptophan, magnesium, and calcium, which aid in melatonin production. If you can't drink milk due to lactose intolerance or another health constraint, you can try replacing it with almond milk or other plant-based milks.

Integrating some of these foods in your diet can be a helpful tool to improve your sleep. However, keep in mind that everyone's body and physiology is different. A food that works very well for one person might not be as helpful to another. If you incorporate any of these foods into your diet, monitor your body's specific response and adjust accordingly.

Foods to Limit before Sleep

While certain foods can help you sleep better, perhaps it's even more important to be aware that others can inhibit your ability to doze off and will have the opposite impact on your sleep. Some foods and beverages consumed too close to bedtime might impair sleep quality and contribute to restless nights. Below is a list of common foods and beverages that you'll likely do better avoiding before bed:

Caffeine:

A well-known and potent stimulant that can keep you awake and attentive for several hours, caffeine before bed can make it harder to fall asleep and remain asleep. Caffeine is not found only in coffee. Other typical sources of caffeine include energy drinks, black, green, and white tea, soda, and even chocolate. I personally try to avoid caffeine for at least six hours before my bedtime to ensure that it does not affect the quality of my sleep. I might make an exception for a low-caffeine food such as a piece dark chocolate, as long as it's a small piece only. But, if someone's body is more sensitive to caffeine, he or she should avoid any caffeine-containing foods for longer, even if only in small quantities.

Alcohol:

Although alcohol may initially induce drowsiness and relaxation, it can impair sleep later in the night. It disrupts your REM sleep, which is crucial for memory and learning. Moreover, alcohol might cause numerous awakenings during the night, resulting in poor sleep quality. Avoid alcohol too close to bedtime to prevent it from interfering with your sleep.

Heavy or Spicy Foods:

Spicy and heavy meals can cause indigestion and heartburn, making it more difficult to fall or remain asleep. Certain foods can also raise your core body temperature, causing you to feel restless and uneasy. It is advisable to avoid heavy foods at least three hours before bedtime to give your stomach adequate time to digest it.

Spices like chili powder, cayenne pepper, and black pepper can raise the body's temperature and cause stomach discomfort and acid reflux. Heavy food and high-fat meals can also cause indigestion making it difficult to fall asleep. The body needs to work harder to digest heavier meals, potentially resulting in discomfort and sleep interruptions. In addition, eating a substantial meal before bedtime can raise the probability of snoring and sleep apnea. Overall, it is advisable to avoid spicy and heavy meals in the evening to encourage better sleep quality. Personally, I avoid these items at least three hours before bedtime. While some individuals may be fine with a shorter time frame than the three hours, others may need to avoid them for even longer to get their optimal sleep.

High Sugar Foods:

Eating foods that are high-in sugar right before bedtime can trigger a sugar spike. This in turn, can lead to a rush of energy that can keep you awake. High sugar foods can also lead to rapid fluctuations in your insulin levels, increasing the risk of diabetes and other metabolic disorders. Avoid foods that are high in sugar for your general wellbeing, and especially avoid them before bedtime if you don't want them to interfere with your rest.

Scheduling of Meals for Better Sleep

It's not just the type of foods that we eat or avoid that can affect our sleep, but the time that we consume them also plays a role. The timing of our last meal of the day can especially be important. As previously said, eating a heavy or spicy meal close to bedtime can cause pain, indigestion, and acid reflux, all of which can impair sleep. Instead, attempt to have dinner at least 2-3 hours before bedtime. If you are hungry and need to eat something later in the evening, then go for a lighter snack that is easy to digest so that it won't interfere with your sleep. A modest bowl of whole-grain cereal with milk or a banana with nut butter are both excellent options. This can also mean not missing meals before dinner which can leave you feeling hungry around night and cause you to have a big meal right before going to bed. Not skipping meals is similar to not skipping water. You should consume sufficient water throughout the day to maintain hydration. Lack of water can have numerous harmful impacts, including making you believe you're hungry and causing you to consume more food. That being said, make sure you're drinking enough water throughout the day so that you don't end up needing to drink too much too close to your bedtime, as too much water right before sleeping might lead you to wake up frequently during the night needing to use the restroom.

Food Allergies and Intolerances:

While many meals can promote or inhibit sleep, it is crucial to note that certain individuals may have food allergies or intolerances that affect their sleep quality differently than other people. When the immune system misidentifies a food as a threat and activates an immunological response, these reactions can occur. This response can cause a variety of symptoms, including digestive difficulties, inflammation, and sleeplessness. It's important to avoid these foods that are causing your problems especially around bedtime.

Gluten Sensitivity

Gluten allergy or sensitivity is a prominent example of a dietary allergy that can affect sleep. Gluten is a protein found in wheat, wheat derivatives, rye, barley and in other grains. In people with celiac disease, gluten allergies, or gluten sensitivity, the consumption of gluten can cause an inflammatory response which in turn can lead to many uncomfortable and painful symptoms. These symptoms may include swelling, hives, shortness of breath, cramps, bloating, diarrhea, and sleep abnormalities. If that's you, you'd want to avoid gluten-containing breads, cereals, grains, crackers, pastas, beers, and other gluten foods. Look for gluten-free options and alternatives.

Lactose Intolerance

Another common example of a food sensitivity is lactose intolerance. People who are lactose intolerance are sensitive to the sugar lactose and will get symptoms from the consumption of milk or other dairy products. These symptoms can include abdominal discomfort, bloating, nausea, indigestion and others. This can provide a good example of how the same food can affect people differently. A small bowl of whole grain cereal with warm milk may be great evening snack for one person that'll help that person relax and fall asleep, while that same bowl of cereal and milk can be a really bad choice for someone with lactose intolerance or a gluten allergy or sensitivity who might instead be all night dealing with symptoms of indigestion, discomfort, and irritability from that meal. That's why it's always important to listen to your body especially as you start trying new approaches and routines.

While gluten and lactose sensitivities may be two of the most common food intolerances that people are aware of, they're far from being the only two. Some of the other frequent food intolerances to be aware of include:

• **Histamine intolerance**: Certain individuals may be sensitive to histamine, a chemical found in specific foods such as aged cheeses, cured meats, and fermented items like yogurt and alcohol. Histamine intolerance can induce headaches, feeling of exhaustion, and sleep difficulties, among other symptoms.

• **Nightshade intolerance**: Nightshades are a group of vegetables that include tomatoes, peppers, potatoes and eggplants. These foods might increase inflammation in some susceptible people. This inflammation can cause joint discomfort, intestinal problems, and sleep disturbances.

• **Caffeine intolerance**: Although it has been indicated that coffee should be avoided a few hours before bedtime, some people may be even more sensitive to its effects and experience sleep disturbances even if they get their caffeine in the early afternoon.

SLEEP LIKE A BABY

In some cases, food intolerances and sensitivities are easy to spot, but in other cases the symptoms can be vague and these food intolerances can go undiagnosed for years leading to persistent symptoms, inflammation, and sleep disturbances. It's therefore important to pay attention to your body and see if there is a connection between the food you eat and how well you sleep or function throughout the day. If you suspect that you might have a food intolerance, you should see a healthcare provider to help you identify the precise triggers and build a plan to avoid them. By doing so, you can enhance your sleep hygiene and your health and well-being. This is also a place where a keeping a sleep diary, one in which you document food eaten throughout the day, can be quite valuable.

A diet rich in whole foods, with adequate amounts of fiber, protein, and nutrients is essential for good health, including healthy sleep patterns. As we have seen in this chapter, certain foods promote sleep while others inhibit it, and the timing of the meals can also affect sleep quality. We can enhance our sleep hygiene and overall health by adopting healthy behaviors such as mindful eating and limiting specific meals before bed. Also, it is important to recognize that there are individual differences, and that those with food allergies or intolerances should avoid trigger foods in order to sleep well. By making minor dietary adjustments and paying attention to how food impacts our sleep, we can attain a more peaceful night's rest and improve the overall quality of our life.

Chapter 5

Stress, Meditation, Yoga and Stretching

Sleep and stress are closely intertwined. Stress can have a detrimental effect on our capacity to fall asleep and stay asleep. This can create a vicious cycle wherein a lack of sleep causes our stress levels to rise even higher, which then results in even worse sleep. Our bodies create more cortisol, a hormone that keeps us awake and alert, while we are under stress. But, if our cortisol levels are regularly high, it may hinder our capacity to get a good night's sleep. Stress may also make it harder for us to calm down and go to sleep since it can make our minds race with worry and anxiety. This can result in a vicious cycle of stress and insufficient sleep, where the latter causes even more stress and cortisol production.

Thankfully, there are several methods we can employ to reduce stress and enhance the quality of our sleep. Stretching, yoga, and meditation are all potent techniques that have been demonstrated to increase relaxation and lower levels of stress. We can increase our capacity to fall asleep fast and stay asleep all night long by routinely using some of these tactics.

In this chapter, we'll go over some of these stress-reduction strategies in greater detail, going over some of their unique sleep advantages and providing advice on how to include them into your daily routine. The objective is not to perfectly implement everything, but by being aware of and implementing some of these strategies, one may notice a significant improvement in their sleep. You can choose the concepts that resonate with you the most. With so many great options and possibilities, pick something you believe you can stick to. These lifestyle adjustments and modifications, like many of the concepts mentioned so far in this book, can have positive effects on your health and fitness beyond just getting enough sleep. Whether you're an experienced yogi or a total novice this section has something for everyone. Let's dive in and see how we can make use of these strategies to promote healthy sleeping habits and lessen the negative effects of stress in our daily life.

Mindful Meditation

Mindfulness meditation is a powerful tool that can help with both stress management and sleep quality. Being mindful entails paying attention to the present moment and accepting one's thoughts, feelings, and experiences without passing judgment. This routine can help us lower our levels of stress and anxiety, promote relaxation, and develop a sense of peace.

You can practice mindful meditation while sitting, lying down, or even going about your everyday business, like folding clothes or cleaning the dishes. The secret is to keep your attention in the here and now while letting go of any distracting ideas or anxieties.

One technique to practice mindful meditation before bed is as follows: Choose a place to sit that is both peaceful and comfortable. You can sit on a chair, or sit cross-legged on the floor, choose whatever position feels more comfortable to you. Close your eyes, take a few long and deep breaths, while focusing on the air going in and out of your body. As you bring your focus on your breathing, you're just watching it without attempting to manipulate it. Notice the air entering, feel your chest and belly rise with each breath, and notice them fall as the breath exits your body. If other thoughts, emotions, and sensations arise, simply acknowledge them, and then bring your attention back to your breath without passing judgment or getting lost in those thoughts. You can also count your breaths by silently counting "one" on the inhale, "two" on the exhale, "three" on the next inhale, and so on, going up to 10 before starting up again. This will help you stay focused on the breath and help prevent your mind from wandering. You may notice that your mind is becoming more relaxed and tranquil as you continue to practice. Continue to refocus your attention on your breath or counting if your mind starts to race. It's crucial to have patience with yourself and not to judge yourself if you start having busy thoughts or find yourself having difficulty keeping your attention on the breathing. Practicing mindful meditation before bed can help you calm your mind and get your body ready for sleep.

Another way to practice mindful meditation is through the use of guided meditation. With guided meditation a calm voice is guiding you through the process reminding you to focus on your breathing and helping you let go of thoughts of distractions. You can find tons of these meditations online and through popular apps available on your phone. You'll find some that are formulated to help with different goals, such as to reduce stress during the day, to help increase self-awareness, or to help improve sleep quality. You'll also find ones of different lengths from a couple of minutes to over an hour long. Choose one that you find soothing and give it a try. Visit HealthMasteryLab.com/sleep for some links and examples.

Studies have shown that mindfulness meditation can significantly improve the quality of sleep and lessen the symptoms of insomnia. It can also have a positive impact on your general mental health.

SLEEP LIKE A BABY

Frequent practice can enhance emotions of satisfaction and wellbeing while reducing stress, anxiety, and depressive symptoms.

Starting slowly and being gentle with oneself are key when you're still new to the practice of mindful meditation. Try to stay consistent, even if it's only a few minutes a day, since consistency is key. With time and effort, mindfulness meditation can become an effective technique and a great instrument in your toolbox that can positively impact your life and your sleep.

There are many forms of meditation other than mindfulness meditation that can enhance the quality of sleep. One such technique is guided imagery, which involves imagining serene and tranquil scenes or scenarios to relax the body and mind. By reducing tension and anxiety, guided imagery can improve sleep. A different form of meditation is the loving-kindness meditation which, as the name suggests, involves concentrating on the feelings of love, kindness, and compassion, toward oneself and toward others. By bringing your attention to these feeling, the practice can elevate one's mood bringing the focus on positive emotions while decreasing stress, which in turn, can promote better sleep. Another popular form of meditation is transcendental meditation. Transcendental meditation makes use of a mantra or other sounds to help calm the mind, lessen tension, and encourage relaxation and better sleep. Transcendental meditation is usually done sitting down in comfortable position.

With the eyes closed you slowly repeat a mantra, such as "Aum", or "Sat Nam" in your head as you try to relax and let go of distracting thoughts. Overall, adopting one or more of these meditation techniques into your nighttime routine can help lower your stress levels, encourage relaxation, and improve you sleep. You can experiment with different forms and find the one that works best for you. Again, start slowly if you have to; if you're new to the practice, your first session doesn't have to be 50 minutes long, instead four or five minutes might be all you need to do to start building this habit and to start experiencing some of the benefits.

Progressive Muscle Relaxation

Progressive muscular relaxation (PMR) is another great strategy for reducing stress and enhancing sleep quality. PMR basically involves tensing up your muscle groups and relaxing them across your body to encourage physical relaxation and help ease muscular tension. You can train your body to relax more readily and deeply by actively tensing and releasing your muscles, which can help lower overall stress levels and enhance sleep.

To practice PMR, find a calm, comfortable spot to sit or lie down with your eyes closed. Start with your feet; tighten the muscles in your feet and toes and hold for a few seconds, then release and completely let go of all the tension in those muscles. Then move up to your ankles and calves and do the same thing, tightening the muscles and holding for a few seconds, then releasing the tension. Work your way slowly up your body going through every muscle group. After the calves move up to the thighs and work your way up through your glutes, lower abdomen, upper abdomen, chest, shoulders, arms, neck, and face. Focus on the tightness and relaxation you feel in each muscle group as you do this and make an effort to let go of any stress or tension you may be harboring.

PMR has been shown to be beneficial in lowering stress and anxiety levels as well as enhancing sleep quality in people suffering from insomnia. It is a wonderful technique that is simple, effective and can be done almost anywhere you can lie down.

Yoga

Yoga is a practice that originated in ancient India but is now practiced all over the world. It has been shown to have great advantages, among which are the benefits of promoting relaxation and decreasing stress. Yoga is an art that combines certain postures with breathing techniques and aspects of meditation. Studies have shown that practicing yoga can have benefits on the quality of sleep. Just like with meditation, there are many different forms of yoga, and going into the details of each form is beyond the scope of this book. However, you do not have to do a full formal yoga session to get all the benefits. Just learning a few positions, like the cobblers' pose or the child's pose and remembering to focus on your breathing can help you get started. Certain forms of yoga, like yoga nidra, incorporates elements of guided meditation in its practice and is often used to help promote a good night sleep.

Adding some elements of yoga in the evening to help promote relaxation can be a great addition to your routing that can help you sleep better. If you're a yoga pro, then that's great, and you should already be using this practice to your advantage. If you've never done it before, but are intrigued, then you can definitely find something useful in learning the practice. Start slow with some of the more gentle positions and with practice you'll be able to advance your technique. There are a lot of available resources that can you get started, from in person classes to online courses and materials, or you can start with some gentle stretching as explained below.

Stretching

Many people who have never practiced yoga before can feel nervous about the idea of taking on this whole new practice that can seem intimidating to them. Other people just don't have the time or space for a comprehensive yoga practice, and others might be unable to perform particular yoga postures due to physical limitations or injuries. If for any reason, you're not interested in yoga at this point, an excellent option is to include some gentle stretching exercises in your nighttime routine. Stretching before bed can aid in easing physical tension, reducing stress, and fostering relaxation, all of which can improve the quality of your sleep. While stretching, paying attention to, and having control of your breathing will also help you unwind both physically and mentally.

There are some easy stretches you can perform before going to sleep. Always pay attention to your body's signals and only do what makes you feel comfortable. Some of these stretches are incorporating some simple yoga positions like the child's pose, while others are simpler stretches that you've probably done at some point in your life before. These mild stretches can be a wonderful place to start for those not interested in a full yoga practice, but still want to reap some of the possible benefits:

(Photos and links to these and similar stretches can be found online at HealthMasteryLab.com/Sleep)

1. Seated Spinal Twist: Sit cross-legged on a mat (or on the floor). Place your left hand on your right knee, and twist to the right, placing your right hand behind you for support. Hold for a few seconds, then switch sides.

2. Child's Pose: On a mat start on your hands and knees. Slowly bring your hip backward as you bend your knees bringing your glutes toward your heels and allowing your arms to stretch. The position should feel very relaxed and comfortable. Relax your head and neck. Take long deep breaths.

3. Butterfly Pose: Sit on the mat, with the soles of your feet touching, forming the butterfly with your legs and knees on the side. You can hold your feet with your arms and comfortably press your knees down toward the floor. Take a few long deep breaths.

4. Standing Forward Fold: You're simply going to stand with your feet hip-width apart and then bend forward toward the ground. Move slowly and gently and do not force yourself or bend more than what you can comfortably do. If you need to bend your knees to avoid discomfort than that's fine. Take a few deep breaths, then gently go back to the standing position.

5. Legs-Up-The-Wall Pose: Lay on your back and stretch your legs up against the wall. You can place a pillow under your hips for support. Like with all other positions you want to be comfortable, and you don't want to force your position.

I also like to incorporate some gentle neck stretches into my evening routine. Remember to always move slowly and gently. You never want to force your neck or body into an uncomfortable or painful positions.

1. Neck Rolls: Sit comfortably with your back straight and with your feet on the floor (or you can sit directly on floor with your legs crossed). The idea is to slowly roll your neck to help release tension. Lower your chin to the chest and roll your neck, gently, to the right side, bringing your right ear and shoulder closer together. Continue rolling to the back so you're looking up and then bringing your left ear toward your left shoulder and back to the starting position. You can start with smaller "rolls" or circles and widen as you go. Repeat a few times, then roll to the other directions for a few times as well.

2. Chin Tucks: Start with your back straight with legs crossed, or feet on floor. As the name suggests, you want to tuck your chin, slowly brining it towards your chest. Keep your shoulders relaxed, hold for a few seconds, then slowly raise it back up. Repeat a few times.

3. Shoulder Shrugs: Sit in the same position with your back straight. Slowly shrug or raise your shoulders up towards your ears, hold for a bit, then relax them back down. Breathe deeply. Repeat a few times.

4. Side Neck Stretches: Sit in a comfortable position with your back straight. You want to bend your neck to the side bringing you ear toward your shoulder one side at a time. You can place your hand, from the same side you're bending toward on top of your head to help gently stretch your neck. Hold for a few seconds on each side, then repeat on the other side.

The stretches listed below may be performed while lying down. I occasionally perform these when lying in bed:

1. Knee-to-Chest Stretch: while lying on your back with your legs extended, slowly start to bring one knee up and towards your chest. Use your hand to gently pull your knee. Hold it there for 10-15 seconds before slowly relaxing your leg back into the extended position and repeating on the other side.

2. Figure Four Stretch: Lie on your back with your knees bent this time. Take one ankle and cross across and over the opposite knee. Pull the bottom bent leg toward your chest. Hold the stretch for 10-15 seconds, then relax gently and switch sides.

3. Spinal Twist: Lie on your back with your knees bent and heels touching. Slowly lower both knees to either side. Try to keep your shoulders relaxed and on the bed. Hold the stretch for 10-15 seconds then rotate back to the starting position. Do the same thing on the other side.

With all the stretches discussed above, always move gently, slowly, and never force yourself into painful or uncomfortable positions. Those stretches should not be strenuous and painful, but rather comfortable and relaxing.

Along with these stretches, incorporating some gentle movements into your nighttime regimen can be helpful. Going for a short walk, trying some Tai Chi, or engaging in another low-impact activity can help promote relaxation. When stretching or doing any other form of gentle exercise, you always want to keep in mind that the type and degree of stretching should be suitable for your individual needs and capabilities; pay attention to your body and avoid pushing yourself too far as excessive or intense stretching can actually have the opposite effect and make it harder to fall asleep.

Remember that the purpose of stretching and light exercise before bed is to assist your body and mind get ready for deep sleep rather than to break a sweat or exhaust yourself. You can find the stretches and movements that are most effective for you with a little experimenting and then include them regularly into your sleep ritual.

The relationship between stress and sleep is bidirectional. While stress can make it harder to fall asleep, the opposite can also be true, and continuous sleep deprivation can increase stress levels in our lives. This vicious cycle can have a nasty effect on the quality of our lives making it harder and harder to fall asleep and harder and harder to enjoy our days.

On the other hand, prioritizing good quality sleep, and reducing stress levels through some of the techniques that we've discussed so far can have wonderful effects on our lives. With better sleep, we're better armed to deal with our daily lives and cope with stressors as they come, and with more peace and less stress throughout the day, we can enjoy a better night's sleep. Living well and having a healthy lifestyle are all interconnected, and by improving one area of our lives through the proper habits and lifestyle modifications, we often see effects of these improvements spilling over into other areas of our lives resulting in better overall well-being.

At the beginning of this chapter, we discussed how stress may result in poorer sleep quality, which can then result in additional stress, producing a negative feedback loop. Instead, we can establish a positive feedback loop that promotes both our physical and mental health by implementing stress management strategies into our daily routines and prioritizing sleep. Through the use of some of these techniques, such as mindfulness meditation, progressive muscle relaxation, yoga, and stretching, we can increase our capacity to control stress, unwind our bodies and minds, and allow ourselves to fall asleep soundly and restoratively.

Chapter 6

Technology and Sleep

Technology is now a part of our daily life that is hard to get away from. While the advantages to technology are so vast, there are some disadvantages that come along with its use as well. One of those disadvantages is the negative effect excessive technology use can have on our sleep. Using one's smartphone and other devices right before bed, or even in bed, is too common a practice. The goal behind this chapter is to provide awareness on how technology, when misused, can negatively affect our sleep, and to discuss some of the things we can do to help mitigate some of these negative effects.

The relationship between sleep and technology has been a hot topic for a number of years. Research has shown how the use of electronic devices before bedtime can have negative consequences on one's ability to sleep restfully affecting both the quantity and the quality of sleep. The blue light emitted for smartphones and television screens for example, can disrupt the body's natural circadian rhythm and inhibit the production of melatonin. In addition to the blue light emitted from the screen, the type of content we're using our screens for also has an effect. If right before going to bed, you decide to scroll through stimulating or anxiety-inducing contents on your phone, whether it's a TV show, the news, or social media posts, and you spend a good amount of time there, chances are, this type of contents will negatively impact your sleep. Additionally, the constant availability of stimulating contents through technology often leaves us in a state of "hyperarousal" where one is always feeling constantly alert and unable to fully relax. This in turn, can affect one's ability to sleep.

Research has also demonstrated that technology use can negatively affect the sleep of children and adolescents. Children can be just as prone, if not more prone, to these negative effects on technology on sleep as are adults. The American Academy of Pediatrics suggests that children and adolescents have a "media curfew" before bed to ensure that they have sufficient time to unwind and prepare for sleep.

SLEEP LIKE A BABY

Minimizing Disruptions from Technology

It's no easy task trying to disconnect from technology on command. Our smartphones are such an integral part of our daily lives nowadays that the idea of going for any certain period of time without one's phone can induce anxiety in many people. Luckily, we don't have to completely abandon technology to be able to get a great night of sleep. However, by implementing a few simple strategies and rules, we can still enjoy the immense benefits our electronic devices bring us, while still minimizing their negative effects on our sleep.

1. Set Technology Boundaries:

Establishing a "media curfew" or a "technology curfew" or a "screen curfew", or whatever you decide to call it can be one of the most effective ways to help limit the negative effects of technology on our sleep. It's a very simple idea, you basically want to set a specific time in the evening after which, the use of screen devices or other electronic devices is not allowed. You can adjust the specifics to whatever make sense to your current situation, but ideally the time you choose to start the media curfew is at least an hour before bedtime, and during that "curfew" all electronic devices such as smartphones, TVs, tablets and laptops are either turned off or set on 'Do Not Disturb' mode. Setting a media curfew is possibly not only a good idea for oneself but can also be a good household rule for the whole family to follow. By disconnecting from screens and stimulating technology before bedtime, your mind will have some time to settle down, unwind and prepare for bed.

2. Use Blue Light Filters:

As we've mentioned in the introduction, the blue light emitted through your television or smartphone screen can disrupt the brain's production of melatonin and your ability to sleep restfully. A simple way to help reduce that exposure is to use a blue light filter. Most smartphones now already come with a built-in setting that'll allow you to adjust your screen's color and reduce blue light exposure. If it's not part of the settings on your device, you can usually find an app that you can download that will help you with blocking the blue light. If you can't find or download the app, you can try blue-light glasses that will filter out and block the blue light from reaching your eyes. This will help restore your natural circadian rhythm and allow you to sleep better.

3. Adjust Device Brightness:

In addition to using blue light filters, it can be beneficial to adjust the brightness of electronic devices. Diminish the brightness of screens in the evening to send the brain the message that it's time to prepare for sleep.

4. Avoid Stimulating Content:

Some types of content can be more stimulating than others, making it more difficult to fall asleep. Avoid watching exciting, suspenseful, or emotionally intense television programs or shows before bed, as these can increase alertness and make it more difficult to unwind.

5. Use "Do Not Disturb" Mode:

Even in silent mode, notifications and alerts from electronic devices can disrupt sleep. Utilize a "Do Not Disturb" mode to muffle notifications during sleep hours.

6. Keep Devices Out of the Bedroom:

It is also advisable to avoid using electronic devices in the bedroom. This can help create an environment conducive to restful sleep, free of technological distractions and disruptions.

Sleep-Friendly Technologies

While it is true that technology can be detrimental to sleep, it can also be used in a variety of ways to promote healthy sleep habits. If you'd like to use technology to your advantage when it comes to your sleep, along with the tips outline above, you can consider some of the following helpful tools:

1. Sleep Tracking Devices:

Sleep tracking devices can track and provide valuable information aspects and characteristics of you sleep. They can track when you went to sleep, when you woke up and how many nighttime awakening you've had. They can also give you other information such as the time spent during each stage of the sleep cycle, your heart rate, your breathing pattern and other pertinent information. This information can give you insight on the quality of your sleep and can be useful to monitor how certain changes you do are affecting the quality of your sleep. These devices are available in many different forms, from smartwatches and wearable rings to smartphone apps and under the mattress tracking devices among others.

2. Smart Lighting:

Smart lights are lights that can be programmed to gradually dim to help simulate a sunset. Many of these lights can also simulate a sunrise in the morning by gradually increasing their intensity. They often come with soothing sounds that can be played in the evening as the light dims to help you relax and go to sleep. The idea is to support your body's circadian rhythm by simulating the sunset pattern in the evening.

3. White Noise Machines:

White noise machines produce a constant, soothing background sound that can help mask out other noises that can disturb your sleep. Those who live in a noisy environment or have trouble falling asleep due to a racing mind may find them particularly useful.

4. Blue Light Filters:

As previously stated, blue light filters can reduce exposure to the blue light emitted by electronic devices. This type of light can interfere with the body's natural melatonin production, making it more difficult to fall asleep. Blue light filters are typically available as apps for mobile devices and tablets, but they can also be purchased as screen protectors and eyeglasses.

5. Sleep Apps:

Numerous sleep apps are available to promote healthy sleep habits, such as apps that provide guided meditations or relaxation exercises to help calm the mind and body before bedtime. Other apps utilize soundscapes or soothing music to aid in relaxation and sleep.

While sleep-friendly technology can be a useful tool for promoting healthy sleep habits, it is important to keep in mind that technology should not be relied on excessively or as the sole remedy for sleep problems. If you choose to utilize any of these apps or tools, you want to do so in conjunction with good sleep hygiene to help you get the optimal results.

Use of Technology by Children and Adolescents

The use of technology among children and adolescents has also increased steadily over the years, and the negative effects excessive technology use can have on sleep are not limited to adults, but can affect children and adolescents as well. As a parent, it's important to set a good example for children and to help direct them and assist them in dealing with these devices so they can form healthy habits that will still allow them to enjoy the benefits of smart technology while still minimizing some of its negative effects on their sleep.

Setting limits on your child's screen time is one way to assist them. Encourage your child to use devices for a limited amount of time each day and set clear rules around when devices can be used and when they should be put away, such as before bedtime. It can also be helpful to establish device-free zones in the house, such as the bedroom, to help your child associate their bedroom with sleep rather than screen time. In addition, parents can encourage their children to participate in activities that promote healthy sleep, such as regular exercise, writing, and spending time outdoors. You can encourage your child to unwind before bed by reading a book, taking a warm bath, or performing gentle stretches. Creating a bedroom environment conducive to sleep with comfortable bedding, dim lighting, and a cool temperature can also improve their quality of sleep.

For adolescents, it is important to educate them on the significance of sleep and the effects of technology on their sleep health. By avoiding the use of electronic devices in the bedroom and establishing a regular sleep routine, they can be encouraged to establish their own healthy sleep habits that would prioritize good rest. It's always helpful to model those habits yourself. Set an example by limiting your own screen time and avoiding technology use before bed. Encourage your adolescent child to engage in nonscreen-based activities, such as playing outside or doing a craft. By establishing healthy technology habits for the whole family, you can help your child get the restful sleep necessary for optimal health and well-being

In conclusion, technology can have significant positive and negative effects on our lives. While technology has brought many benefits to our lives, it has also introduced sleep-disrupting obstacles. By understanding the connection underlying the relationship between technology and sleep, we can take measures to mitigate some of these negative effects and promote healthy sleep habits.

Utilizing blue light filters, avoiding screen time before bed, and creating a bedroom environment conducive to sleep are great methods for minimizing disruptions caused by technology use. You can also consider sleep-friendly technology, which consists of tools and devices designed to encourage healthy sleeping habits.

Each individual is different, and some people are going to be more sensitive to screen use and other technologies before bedtime, while for the others, the effects won't be as significant. In terms of implementing some of the strategies we've talked about, that will also be easier for some than others. You may already incorporate some of these techniques in your life, or maybe it's all new to you. If you find it difficult to implement some of these strategies, you can start by taking smaller steps toward the goal in mind. For example, you can set a media curfew that's only 15 minutes prior to your sleep and then increase the time by increments until you get to your goal. Technology and screens are now a part of our daily life, but it's still important to be aware of some of their unintended negative side effects so that we can take steps to help mitigate them and give us ourselves the best shot at getting the restful sleep we require.

You can look the resource section of the book for links to some of the technologies discussed here. As these devices are constantly being updated, we'll be able to update the list regularly on the website.

Chapter 7

Natural Remedies for sleep

People have been using and relying on herbal remedies for ages. These remedies are vast in number and can have many different roles including promoting relaxation and aiding in restful sleep. While those remedies are not a guaranteed solution for everyone with significant and persistent insomnia, they can be the missing piece for some individuals, and many will find them as a helpful addition to their sleep routine. Herbal remedies com in many forms; you can find them as teas, capsules, tinctures, and essential oils. In this chapter, we will take a look at some of the most popular and commonly used herbs for sleep, and we'll talk about how they might be utilized to promote a more restful night's rest.

Although the full mechanism by which herbal treatments can improve sleep are not completely understood, we have many ideas about some of the ways in which they can positively affect our sleep cycle. Certain herbs are likely to increase the production of GABA, a specific neurotransmitter that plays a major role in relaxing and calming our nervous system. Some herbs have molecules that can directly interact with certain brain receptors resulting in a calming effect as well. Other herbs might work by helping regulate our circadian rhythm or normalize certain stress hormones like cortisol Ashwagandha likely falls in that category. There are probably many more ways that are not yet fully understood by which these supplements can interact with our bodies and nervous system and cause their effects. What we do know however, is that certain herbal remedies can help us improve our sleep quality and quantity.

While herbal remedies are generally safe, they can in some people cause side effects, especially if taken in really high doses above the typical recommendations. This is especially true for people who already have a sensitive digestive system, are under the care of a physician for chronic medical conditions or are taking other medications that might possibly interact with these herbal remedies. So, use good judgement, and consult with your doctor before starting any new regimen, especially if you're taking other medications or have other health concerns.

Herbal remedies come in many different forms, such tablets, capsules, tinctures, essential oils, and others. Yet, one of the most common and well-known methods to consume these remedies is through herbal teas. Making a cup of herbal tea is a simple and straightforward method for enjoying the benefits of these natural treatments. For many herbs, this simply involves steeping them in boiling water for 5 to 10 minutes before straining and enjoying. Nevertheless, some will require different preparation methods, so be careful to read and adhere to the instructions for each herb you purchase. Tinctures and essential oils are also common ways to use these remedies, however preparation may be required. Tinctures are concentrated herbal extracts that, depending on how they are made, can be added to teas or consumed orally. Essential oils can be diffused or applied topically. We'll have a whole chapter on essential oils next.

Chamomile:

Chamomile, a well-known plant with relaxing effects, is one of the most widely used teas to help with sleep and relaxation. Chamomile is native to Europe and Asia and is a member of the daisy family. German chamomile (Matricaria chamomilla) and Roman chamomile (Chamaemelum nobile) are the two common varieties of chamomile Both varieties can be used for their relaxing and soothing effects. Often, you'll find German chamomile being used to treat digestive disorders and inflammation, whilst Roman chamomile is more known to be used for relaxation and sleep.

One way to use chamomile is to prepare it as tea. You can simply steep dried chamomile flowers (or fresh chamomile if you have it) in boiling water for several minutes. Chamomile tea is also readily available in supermarkets and can be easily prepared at home. A small cup at night can be tried to help induce relaxation and enhance your sleep quality.

You can find chamomile in other forms as well, such as capsules, tinctures, and essential oils. Capsules and tinctures may be used orally, whilst essential oils may be applied topically or utilized in aromatherapy.

Valerian Root

Native to Europe and Asia, valerian root has been utilized for ages for its soothing qualities. It is frequently employed as a natural cure for insomnia and other sleep-related problems. Valerian root contains sedative chemicals, and studies indicates that it can enhance sleep quality and help individuals fall asleep faster. It is thought that valerian root is particularly useful for people who suffer from anxiety and sleep difficulties caused by stress.

Typically, Valerian root is found in the form of capsules, pills, liquid extracts, or teas. Some individuals dislike the scent of valerian root, which is why it is commonly used in capsule or tablet form. Because the potency and purity of valerian root products can vary greatly, it is essential to obtain it from a trusted supplier.

SLEEP LIKE A BABY

Lavender

Lavender is another herb that has been long used for its relaxing and soothing effects. It is well-known for its sweet scent and lovely purple blooms. Native to the Mediterranean, the plant is now farmed globally.

Lavender is frequently used to help induce relaxation and restful sleep. Terpenes, a class of aromatic molecules present inside the plant, are at least partly responsible for lavender's sedative properties. It is thought that these substances interact with the neurological nervous system and induce serenity and relaxation, hence enhancing sleep quality. According to studies, lavender can lower anxiety, enhance the quality of sleep, and promote sensations of relaxation.

Lavender may be utilized in a variety of ways to improve sleep. Lavender essential oil, which may be diffused in a room or added to a warm bath, is one of the most typical methods. You can also find lavender-scented pillows online. Lavender is also available as tea, powder, and capsules.

Passionflower

Passionflower is yet another plant that have been used for many generations to help people sleep better and as a remedy for stress and anxiety. Native to the Americas, the use of the Passionflower plant dates all the way back to the Aztecs. The plant is an exquisite, ornamental vine with beautiful, colorful flowers. Its scientific name is Passiflora incarnata, but it also has other cultural names including maypop, apricot vine, and wild passion vine. The plan can grow up to 30 feet high and it's leaves and stems are what's often used to produce passionflower products and extracts.

Passionflower is believed to help relax the mind and reduce symptoms of anxiety. Therefore, it can also be used as a helpful sleep remedy, especially for those suffering from too many thoughts before bed. It likely has direct sedative effects on the nervous system which is how it can help a person fall asleep faster. The plant is available in many forms including tablets, capsules, tinctures and teas. Passionflower tea is a common and a popular beverage consumed worldwide and is usually readily available in stores and online.

Lemon Balm

Lemon Balm is a plant from the mint family. Its leaves are short and green, and its small flowers are usually either white or yellow. It can grow year-round, and it's grown all over the world. Its scientific name is Melissa officinalis, and it has a pleasant lemony scent. It has a long history of use in herbal medicine, due to its calming and relaxing properties, including use in those suffering from sleep difficulties. Lemon balm contains compounds like eugenol and rosmarinic acid, a polyphenol, which are natural compounds that have sedative qualities and can wield a relaxing effect on the mind and body.

In addition to promoting relaxation and reducing anxiety, which might enhance sleep quality, lemon balm can also enhance mood. This may be particularly beneficial for people who have trouble sleeping due to feelings of sadness or worry. Lemon balm is available in capsules, tablets, or as a tea or an essential oil. Lemon balm tea can usually be prepared by steeping the fresh or dried leaves in boiling water for about five to ten minutes.

There is a multitude of other herbs that have been long used to help promote relaxation and to help people fall asleep faster. While chamomile, valerian root, lavender, passionflower, and lemon balm are some of the most well-known ones, other examples include:

Hops are the blossoms of the hop plant, which have historically been used to flavor beer. Yet, hops contain sedative effects and have been used as a natural sleep aid for ages. Hops can be used as a tea, tincture, or capsule and are frequently mixed with other herbs, such as valerian root, for a stronger impact. Hops are thought to promote relaxation and mental calmness, making it easier to fall asleep.

Skullcap is a blooming plant that is indigenous to North America. It has long been used to treat anxiety and nervous disorders, and it is considered to possess sedative characteristics that make it beneficial for promoting good quality sleep. Skullcap can be used as a tea or tincture, and is frequently mixed with other herbs, such as valerian root or passionflower, to increase its potency. It is thought that skullcap facilitates sleep by calming the mind and promoting relaxation.

Kava is a native South Pacific plant that has long been used as a ceremonial beverage for its calming and relaxing qualities. It has been discovered that kava has sedative qualities and is frequently used to encourage sleep and alleviate anxiety. Kava may be used as a tea, pill, or tincture, and it is thought to operate by raising GABA levels, a neurotransmitter that promotes relaxation and tranquility.

Ashwagandha is a plant widely used in Ayurveda medicine for its adaptogenic effects, and its ability to alleviate stress and anxiety. While historically not considered a sleep aid, ashwagandha has been proven to possess sedative qualities and may help promote relaxation which can in turn enhance sleep quality. Ashwagandha can be used as a tea, capsule, powder, or tablet, and is frequently mixed with other herbs, such as valerian root or passionflower, to increase its potency.

Mixing Herbal Treatments for Better Sleep

There are various advantages to combining herbs, as that can enhance their unique properties and provide a synergistic impact that may be stronger than utilizing a single plant alone. By mixing valerian root with hops or passionflower, for instance, the calming properties of each herb can be amplified, resulting in deeper relaxation and greater sleep. Similarly, mixing chamomile with lavender can have a more soothing impact on the mind and body, lowering anxiety, stress, and tension. Several herbal products you'll find at the grocery store already contain these and other herbal combinations. There is no one right answer for everybody. Some people will prefer the combination products while some prefer to use pure single ingredient products. Note that not all herbs should be blended, so use caution if you're making your own blend and do the appropriate research first.

While these herbs are generally considered safe, some individuals can experience side effects from their use especially if taken in large quantities. Whenever you add a new herb, supplement or remedy to your routine, you want to pay attention to your body and see how you're personally reacting to it. Keep track of your sleep pattern after trying one of these remedies to see if it's working for you, or if you need to adjust. A sleep diary is not necessary, but it can be a helpful tool to track your progress. Most individuals can tolerate those herbs extremely well, but it's still crucial to talk to your healthcare provider before adding any supplements to your diet, especially if you are taking any prescriptions, are pregnant or nursing, or have any underlying medical conditions or concerns.

Chapter 8

Aromatherapy and Sleep

Aromatherapy, which refers to the use of essential oils to boost physical and mental health, is a practice that has been around for centuries. It has been used for multiple purposes, among which are promoting relaxation and improving sleep. Essential oils are highly concentrated plant extracts containing the natural aromatic components responsible for the fragrance and medicinal capabilities of the plant.

In recent years, the use of essential oils as a natural alternative to pharmaceutical sleep aids has gained popularity. Essential oils can be inhaled, used topically, or used in a diffuser to promote peaceful sleep by creating a calming environment. Essential oils include natural components that can interact with the limbic system, which regulates emotions and actions. Essential oil inhalation can activate the olfactory system, triggering a relaxation response and promoting sensations of peace and relaxation. Thus, it is thought that those essential oils function by inducing a state of relaxation and serenity that aids in sleep. Essential oils also contain a class of chemicals and compounds that are calming in nature and have that soothing effect on the body that can facilitate better sleep by enabling the body and mind to relax.

Essential oil can be utilized in a variety of methods, including their use through a diffuser, topical application, and inhalation.

Diffusing

The use of a diffuser is one of the most common ways to utilize essential oils and enjoy their benefits. A diffuser is a device that scatters essential oils into the air as a fine mist or vapor, allowing you to inhale the scent and benefit from its therapeutic properties. There are many types of diffusers you can find online, but the four most common ones are ultrasonic, nebulizing, thermal, and evaporative.

As the name suggests, ultrasonic diffusers make use of ultrasonic vibrations as their main mechanism of dispersing the essential oil particles into a thin mist and diffusing it into the air. This type of diffuser is popular since it is both silent and simple to use. Some ultrasonic diffusers have LED lights, which can create a relaxing atmosphere in your bedroom.

Nebulizing diffusers utilize pressured air to disperse essential oils as a thin mist into the air. This type of diffuser is often more costly than ultrasonic diffusers, but it is incredibly effective at diffusing the oils and producing a powerful scent.

Heat diffusers disperse essential oils into the air using heat. This type of diffuser is affordable and simple to use, however it may not disperse essential oils as effectively as ultrasonic and nebulizing diffusers. In addition, heat can change the chemical makeup of some oils, diminishing their medicinal value.

Using a fan or other mechanical device, evaporative diffusers blow air across a pad or filter saturated with essential oils. This allows the essential oils to evaporate and generate a fragrance in the air. This sort of diffuser is generally affordable and simple to use, however it may not disperse essential oils as effectively as other options.

Typically, all you need to do to use a diffuser is to fill the reservoir with water and add a few drops of your preferred essential oil. Then, activate the diffuser and allow it to run for a specified period of time, often between 30 minutes and two hours. However, it is crucial to follow the instructions included with your diffuser, since the precise amount of water and essential oil and the time required may vary depending on the device. Moreover, ensure that the diffuser you select is adequate for the size of the space in which it will be used. For instance, a bigger diffuser is advised for a living room or a bedroom, whilst a smaller one is appropriate for a bathroom or a small workplace.

It is important to use high-quality, pure essential oils when employing a diffuser. Cheaper and synthetic oils may include compounds that are harmful when breathed. Also, make sure you use an oil that aligns with your specific needs. Always do your research and consult a health professional if needed before starting a new regimen.

Topical Application

With topical application, you're applying the essential oil preparation (after properly diluting it) directly onto the skin. Because the oils are absorbed into your blood circulation through your skin, their therapeutic characteristics can have an influence on the entire body and not just on the area where they applied. Topical application of the right oils in the right mixture can be very useful for encouraging relaxation and facilitating sleep.

To apply essential oils topically, it's important to first prepare them by diluting them with a carrier oil such as jojoba oil, coconut oil, or almond oil. Essential oils are often too powerful for direct application to the skin. Diluting the oils prevents skin irritation and sensitization.

To produce a topical mixture, thoroughly combine a few drops of the essential oil of your choosing with a carrier oil. Once mixed and ready to use, focus on regions such as the neck, temples, wrists, and soles of the feet when applying. You can also massage the mixture into the skin which can help with the absorption of the oils.

Be aware that certain essential oils can be photosensitive, which means that they can cause skin irritation or discoloration when exposed to sunlight. Bergamot, grapefruit, and lemon oils are all examples of photosensitive oils. Thus, it is advised to avoid using these oils topically before going outdoors during the day and use them at night instead.

Also, it is vital to always do a patch test prior to using a new essential oil, since some people may be allergic or sensitive to specific oils. To do a patch test, dilute the essential oil with a carrier oil and apply a little amount to a small area of skin, such as the inside of the arm. Wait 24 hours to evaluate whether irritation or sensitivity develops before using the oil in larger quantities.

Inhalation

Inhalation is another method for utilizing essential oils for sleep. When inhaled, the scent of the oils can activate the olfactory system in the brain, therefore promoting relaxation and enhancing sleep quality. You can use a diffuser as already mentioned, which technically is a method of inhalation, or you utilize steam inhalation or direct inhalation.

Steam inhalation consists of adding a few drops of the essential oil to a bowl of hot water, covering the head with a towel, and breathing the steam. This approach is especially useful for cleaning the sinuses and decreasing congestion, both of which can cause sleep difficulties.

With direct inhalation, a few drops of the essential oil are placed on a tissue or cotton ball, and the aroma is then inhaled from there This technique can be quick and handy, but it may not be as successful as other techniques for promoting relaxation and enhancing sleep.

It is critical to highlight that essential oils should never be inhaled directly from the container, since they can be too concentrated and therefore, possibly harmful. Follow the directions on the bottle when trying a new oil, and always start small and increase appropriately as needed.

Commonly Used Essential Oil

With so many different essential oil options on the market, it can be a little overwhelming for someone just starting out. While there are many, a few do stand out in a class of their own. Some of the most well-known and commonly used essential oils for sleep and relaxation include:

Lavender

Probably the most well-known essential oil for sleep improvement, lavender has a lovely, floral scent that is known for its ability to induce a state of calmness and relaxation. Research has shown that lavender use can enhance the quality of sleep in people suffering with insomnia, while also reducing anxious and depressive symptoms. It's probably through its calming and soothing effects, that lavender helps people sleep quicker. To use lavender, you can place a few drops in an essential oil diffuser, add it to a warm bath, or use the inhalation or topical method.

Chamomile

Chamomile is another very well-known essential oil that can help promote sleep. We've already mentioned chamomile in the natural remedies section and spoke about its benefits when used as an herbal tea. It also comes as an essential oil and can also be used that way to help promote a restful sleep. The oil has a gentle, calming scent that can promote feeling of calmness and relaxation and sooth the mind. Chamomile is known for its sedative properties and ability to reduce stress and anxiety. These properties make it a great option for many who are looking for an herbal remedy or an essential oil they can use to help them with their sleep. Additionally, chamomile likely has some pain-relief properties, which can be particularly useful if physical discomfort also plays a role in one's insomnia. As an essential oil, chamomile can be used in a diffuser, added to a warm bath, or through one of the other methods we've discussed.

Bergamot

Derived from the peels of the bergamot orange, bergamot essential oil is known to have a refreshing calming sense. Bergamot essential oil contains natural compounds, such as linalool and limonene, which are believed to have soothing effects on the mind. Because it can promote a feeling of relaxation and decrease feelings of stress, it's often used as a natural sleeping aid. Bergamot, however, can have photosensitizing properties, and cause skin irritations on some individuals, especially if applied topically and then exposed to the sun. It can be a great essential oil to use for sleep, but always test it first and use in the proper diluted form.

Ylang-ylang

Ylang-ylang essential oil is derived from the blooms of the Southeast Asian Cananga odorata tree. It is considered to have a relaxing and sedative impact on the body and mind, with its pleasant and flowery scent. Traditionally, ylang-ylang essential oil has been utilized as a natural cure for anxiety and stress, making it an excellent choice for encouraging relaxation and improving sleep. Its aroma has also been demonstrated to lower blood pressure and heart rate. Before bed, ylang-ylang essential oil can be diffused or applied topically to the chest, wrists, or soles of the feet with a carrier oil. It mixes nicely with other soothing oils, such as lavender and chamomile, to help enhance their calming effects.

Valerian

Valerian is a potent essential oil that has been used to aid in relaxation for generations. Its calming effects make it a good choice for insomnia and anxiety. Valerian oil is extracted from the root of the Valeriana officinalis plant and has a powerful, earthy odor that some individuals can find too strong. Yet, when taken in modest doses or in combination with other essential oils, valerian can increase the quality and length of sleep. It can be diffused, added to a bath, or administered topically in a carrier oil to promote deep sleep and relaxation. Nonetheless, due to its strength, it is advised to use valerian oil sparingly and start with a small amount only.

Cedarwood oil

Due to its grounding and relaxing characteristics, cedarwood essential oil can be excellent for supporting better sleep in some individuals. It is well-known for its woody, warm, and somewhat sweet perfume, which can help create a tranquil and restful atmosphere in the bedroom. It is derived from coniferous trees around the world and has been used for ages. Cedarwood oil is thought to have sedative effects as well as the ability to reduce stress and anxiety, and both properties can make it a great choice to help one fall asleep faster and reduce nighttime awakenings. Cedarwood essential oil can be used in a diffuser, through topical application or through steam inhalation.

Sandalwood

This is another oil that has been used for generations to help promote better sleep and calmness. Obtained from certain species of the sandalwood trees, this oil has a warm woody aroma that can soothe the mind and relax the body. Sandalwood is believed to at least partly work through having effects on the limbic system, the portion of the brain that regulates emotions and actions, and balancing the body's natural cycles. Because it may aid in reducing anxiety and promoting feelings of calmness, it can be a perfect choice for some people who battle with racing thoughts before their sleep. To use, you can add a few drops to a diffuser, use steam inhalation, or dilute and apply topically.

Vetiver

Vetiver essential oil is renowned for its relaxing and grounding effects. This earthy-smelling oil is derived from the roots of the Vetiver plant. Vetiver oil is frequently used to help relax the mind and lessen feelings of tension or stress, which can make falling asleep and staying asleep easier. It can be diffused or used topically prior to bedtime to encourage a restful night's sleep.

Clary sage

Clary sage is another essential oil that is frequently used to promote relaxation. It has a warm, earthy, and somewhat sweet aroma that can aid in calming the mind and reducing worry or tension. It has sedative properties that can help promote sleep. You can use it in a diffuser or through steam inhalation or topical application. Using clary sage before bed can possibly lower blood pressure and decrease the heart rate which can help calm the body. Be aware that clary sage, however, can cause drowsiness in some people, so use cautiously and don't use before driving or if operating heavy machinery.

Marjoram

Marjoram, which is often used as a food additive, is also found as an essential oil and can have benefits on promoting good quality sleep. Its essential oil has a warm, soothing aroma that can help ease anxious feelings and promote relaxation, allowing for better sleep. Some studies suggest that Marjoram can help regulate breathing patterns, which may make it particularly useful for those who struggle with snoring during their sleep or sleep apnea. It's a great essential oil to try, and can be used in a diffuser, through topical application, or through steam inhalation.

Patchouli

Patchouli essential oil comes from the leaves of the patchouli plant, a plant native to the tropical parts of Asia. It has a deep, earthy scent and it is a popular option in certain parts of the world as a sleep promoting product. With its strong musky aroma, Patchouli is believed to have some sedative effects while also being able to help relax the mind and decrease feelings of tension and anxiety. When used in a diffuser or through steam inhalation it can help create a sense of calm and peace that can help promote deep sleep.

Frankincense

Frankincense is a versatile essential oil that has been utilized for generations due to its relaxing and grounding effects. It is extracted from the Boswellia tree's resin and has a woody, spicy, and somewhat sweet scent. The ability of frankincense essential oil to induce relaxation, reduce anxiety, and calm the mind makes it a great option for supporting a restful sleep. Frankincense is also widely used for its anti-inflammatory effects as well and may be particularly useful in those suffering from inflammatory issues. A few drops of frankincense essential oil can be added to a diffuser or blended with the appropriate carrier oil and applied to the skin.

Neroli

Neroli essential oil is derived from the bitter orange tree's blooms. Neroli is a popular choice in aromatherapy for sleep due to its pleasant, flowery scent, which can encourage relaxation and reduce anxiety. It is thought that the essential oil is able to interact with the limbic system, resulting in its soothing effects over the mind. It's also believed that Neroli can lower chronic inflammation in the body. It can be used through a diffuser, steam inhalation or topical application to help promote a relaxing environment and encourage a good night's sleep.

In addition to the previously discussed essential oils, there are several additional oils that may be used to help induce sleep. An example is jasmine essential oil, with its sweet and flowery scent, which is recognized for its relaxing and sedative qualities. Rose essential oil also has a pleasant and flowery aroma that can encourage relaxation and reduce anxiety, making it a great choice for enhancing sleep as well. There are many more options you can explore if you're more interested in the field, but the ones mentioned so far are a great place to start.

Essential Oils to Consider Avoiding

While the right essential oils can be great at promoting sleep and relaxation, other essential oils should be avoided before bedtime since they have the opposite effect and can potentially disturb sleep. I would avoid the following essential oils before bed:

Citrus oils, such as lemon, lime, and grapefruit oils, are renowned for their uplifting and revitalizing qualities. While these essential oils may be beneficial throughout the day, they may be too stimulating before night and make it more difficult to fall asleep.

Peppermint oil is frequently used for its refreshing and reviving properties; however, it might be overly stimulating before night and interfere with sleep.

Rosemary oil may help memory and topically it can possibly aid in hair growth. It also can be too revitalizing and stimulating before bedtime and interrupt sleep.

Eucalyptus oil: Eucalyptus oil is often used for respiratory disorders and can be beneficial during the day, but its strong aroma can be overbearing before bedtime and may disrupt sleep.

Cinnamon oil has a strong, spicy aroma that may be too stimulating before bedtime and impair sleep.

Thyme essential oil is renowned for its invigorating and revitalizing effects. It is frequently used to enhance attention and concentration, making it a better choice for daytime use than before bedtime.

Pine essential oil with its fresh, woody, and energizing aroma can help enhance concentration and alertness. As a result, it is frequently employed in aromatherapy to battle fatigue and enhance mental clarity. Hence, it may be better used during the day and not right before sleep.

Tea tree essential oil is frequently used in skin care and cleaning products due its antibacterial and antifungal characteristics; however, it is not generally utilized for encouraging relaxation and sleep due to its stimulating effect on the mind and body.

It is important to remember that everyone's reaction to essential oils may vary. Some may find that a specific oil works very well for their sleep while others may find that the same oil not as useful, but the above guidelines can be a great place to start. Experiment with several oils to see which one works best for you, but exercise caution when testing new oils, especially before bed.

Essential Oil Blends for Sleep

In addition to utilizing individual essential oils for sleep and relaxation, blending oils can enhance their specific qualities and produce a more effective impact Combining essential oils will allow you to customize your blend to your specific preferences and needs, allowing for an individualized approach.

With a diffuser, you can blend two to three drops of lavender, chamomile, and bergamot essential oils. These oils are all well-known for their calming and relaxing characteristics and can work well together to help create a soothing environment conducive to sleep. Combining lavender, ylang-ylang, and cedarwood, all of which have comforting tranquil effects as well, is another blend I frequently use. On occasion, I enjoy mixing frankincense, clary sage, and marjoram as a stress-relieving blend to help calm the nerves and alleviate tension. Vetiver, sandalwood, and patchouli can work nicely together, and I frequently use that combination as a calming blend, particularly when my mind seems scattered. Depending on one's preferences, there are so many other mixtures one can try. Trying to find oils of complimentary characteristics and mixing them together to create a superior blend for relaxation or anxiety reduction and sleep improvement can both be a joyful and a rewarding process. I personally use most of these blends in a diffuser, but you can also make blends for topical applications as well. If you make a new topical mix, make sure you're adequately diluting it in the proper carrier oil, and start with a test spot first. Always make sure you're choosing high quality oils from a reliable source to ensure their efficacy and their safety.

Essential oils are plant extracts with natural compounds that, when used properly, can have a number of benefits on our sleep and our wellbeing. Nonetheless, it's important to use them appropriately and safely to avoid potential side effects. Certain essential oils might cause adverse reactions, especially when they are used improperly or in excess. For instance, if not adequately diluted, certain essential oils can cause skin irritation and hypersensitivity. Others, such eucalyptus and peppermint, might irritate the respiratory system when breathed in high doses. Before using essential oils, it is important to do your research on their proper use and potential side effects, and to always adhere to the suggested dilution ratios and usage instructions. Pregnant women and small children should always exercise extra caution when using essential oils. During pregnancy, some essential oils, such as clary sage and sage, should be avoided since they might trigger uterine contractions. Before using essential oils, anyone with medical issues or taking medications should first consult with their healthcare provider.

In general, essential oils are a safe and efficient method for promoting health and well-being. Nonetheless, it is essential to use them in a safe and responsible manner to avoid any problems or side effects. Always do your research and dilute correctly. Exercise caution, especially when used in pregnant women, small children, or if you have any medical conditions or are taking medications.

By including essential oils into your bedtime ritual, you can create a tranquil and relaxing environment conducive to a sound and restful sleep. It has been shown that the usage of essential oils can help reduce tension and anxiety, improve breathing patterns, and promote a deeper, more restful sleep.

There are several resources available if you are interested in learning more about essential oils for sleep or experimenting with different mixtures. For further information, you can speak with a qualified aromatherapist or visit the online resources page at HealthMasteryLab.com/Sleep for further information.

Chapter 9

Homeopathic Remedies for Sleep

Homeopathy as a field was originated by Samuel Hahnemann, a German physician, in the late 18th century as a form of alternative medicine. It was based on the belief that "like heals like," meaning that a drug that creates symptoms in a healthy individual may be used to treat those same symptoms in a sick one, but the field has developed and evolved since then. Homeopathic remedies are often extremely diluted, frequently to the point where there is little or no active component remaining in the preparation and are said to work by stimulating the body's intrinsic healing capabilities.

Homeopathy has been utilized for more than two centuries and has been attaining increased recognition and popularity, with practitioners and clinics found worldwide. In some areas, like certain parts of India, homeopathy is considered mainstream medicine and practiced extensively. However, due to the absence of scientific proof for its usefulness and the extremely diluted nature of the medicines, it remains controversial in many medical circles. Still, despite this controversy, many people continue to utilize homeopathic medicines for a range of health ailments, including sleep problems. Some individuals favor homeopathy because they see it as a natural and holistic approach to medicine, and they value the personalized approach homeopaths often use when selecting medications, basing it on an individual's unique symptoms and health history. Therefore, it can be worth learning about these homeopathic remedies, and trying them for oneself, especially that many do exist to help address sleep problems.

Homeopathic sleep aids come in many forms, including pills, pellets, liquids, and topical treatments. Tablets are the most popular type and are often dissolved under the tongue. Some liquid preparations can be mixed with water, while others can be consumed undiluted. When taking homeopathic medicines for sleep, it is crucial to adhere to the prescribed dosage and frequency as specified on the product label or as instructed by a homeopathic practitioner. Generally speaking, these remedies are taken at least 30 minutes prior to bedtime, and it's usually advised to refrain from consuming anything else other than water during that time. Before beginning a new therapy, it is always important to contact a healthcare professional because certain homeopathic treatments may interfere with other drugs or supplements.

Here are some of the most often utilized homeopathic treatments for sleep:

Coffea Cruda

This remedy, derived from unroasted coffee beans, is frequently used to help insomnia caused by a hyperactive mind or excessive enthusiasm. Coffea cruda, despite it being manufactured from coffee beans, is not a stimulant and is not consumed for its caffeine content. Rather, it is thought to regulate and restore the body's normal sleep-wake cycle on a subtle energy level. Typically, coffea cruda is consumed as a pellet dissolved beneath the tongue.

Nux Vomica

Nux vomica is derived from the seeds of the strychnine tree and is sometimes used as a homeopathic treatment for insomnia. This remedy is one of the more controversial ones as people can suffer potential side effects from this treatment, so be cautious and talk to your primary care provider before starting this one.

Chamomilla

This treatment, derived from chamomile flowers, is frequently used to alleviate sleeplessness brought on by mental stress or physical discomfort. The chamomile plant has been a consistent theme in this book because of its multiple possible benefits on sleep as previously discussed.

Pulsatilla

This treatment is derived from the windflower and is frequently used to treat insomnia brought on by hormonal fluctuations, such as those that occur during menstruation or menopause. Those who have problems sleeping due to a sense of being too hot or too chilly may also benefit.

Passiflora

This passionflower-derived medicine is frequently used to alleviate insomnia induced by worry or tension. Those who wake up frequently during the night may also benefit.

Kali-Phos

This potassium phosphate-based medication is frequently used to treat insomnia caused by mental or emotional distress. It can also be beneficial for people who have difficulty falling asleep due to anxiety or excessive thought.

In addition to individual homeopathic remedies for sleep, combination treatments are also available for purchase. These combination homeopathic sleep aids typically combine multiple remedies into a single product, often providing a more potent approach to the problem.

Combination remedies offer the advantage of a possibly more potent and targeted approach while still being convenient and easy to use. However, the drawbacks to available combination treatments include the limited ability to customize as well as the potential for side effects and interactions. Combination therapies can work very well for some people but not as well for others. When selecting a therapy, make sure you choose the right one for your particular needs; for example, some are formulated to help you sleep faster, while others are designed more to target anxiety and restlessness. Always read the instructions on the label for proper use, and if you're unsure or have any questions, make sure you consult with an expert first. Common combination therapies for sleep include Hyland's Calms, Bach Rescue Sleep, and Boiron Quietude.

Most homeopathic remedies are very diluted forms of the active ingredient and are generally safe. Side effects, however, can and do occur. Always use safely, and check with you healthcare provider before starting a new regimen, especially if you're pregnant, breastfeeding, are taking medications or have any medical issues or concerns. Also make sure you monitor your body's response to the treatment to see if it's working for you or if you need to adjust.

In conclusion, homeopathic remedies are generally a safe option, and many people like to use them as an alternative to other pharmaceutical treatments. The research on many of these remedies is still limited, but their use is quite popular, and many people do report positive outcomes with them. If you decide to give these remedies a try, make sure you're doing it safely and responsibly, and monitor your response to see if it's working for you so that you can adjust accordingly. A well-trained homeopathic practitioner can help guide you along the way and help give you more advice if needed. The Resources page at HealthMasteryLab.com/sleep will also have additional information if you're interested more in the subject.

Chapter 10

Supplements for Sleep

Supplement use is becoming a more common practice. Supplements is a broad category that can refer to a variety of products that may include vitamins, minerals, amino acids, herbs, or other dietary ingredients, that are meant to provide benefits to one's wellbeing supplementing their diet. They can help address a wide variety of health issue, and a large number of supplements available are meant to address sleep concerns. For example, some sleep aid supplements may contain specific vitamins and minerals that help normalize the body's sleep-wake cycle, or they may help regulate the synthesis of hormones that regulate mood and sleep, like serotonin. Supplements come in many forms, from tablets and capsules, which are among the most common, to liquids, powders, or even serums and lotions for topical use. Talk to your physician before starting a new supplement, especially if you're pregnant, are taking medications, or have any medical issues or concerns. Below, we will discuss the most prevalent supplements for sleep:

Melatonin

Melatonin is probably the most well-known of the sleep supplements. It's a hormone that is produced by the pineal gland and one of its main functions is to help regulate the body's circadian rhythm. Naturally, melatonin levels fall in the morning and rise at night. The rising levels of melatonin at night help signal to the brain that's it's time to wind down and get ready to sleep. Therefore, it's no surprise that melatonin is often used to help people go to sleep as an increase in its levels, through supplementation, can help tell the body that it's time to relax and prepare for sleep. This can be especially helpful in people who have difficulties making sufficient melatonin, which may result in problems going to sleep or remaining asleep throughout the night.

As a supplement melatonin can assist in regulating the circadian rhythm and enhancing the quality of your sleep. You can get melatonin over the counter in a variety of forms, from pills and capsules, to gummy bears and liquid solutions. Individual characteristics such as age, weight, and the severity of the sleep disorder can all influence the required dosage of melatonin, but in general, a dosage of 0.5-2 mg of melatonin is common among adults. You usually want to a start with a smaller dose and gradually increase it as necessary. Also, it is advisable to take melatonin tablets 30 to 60 minutes before bedtime to give the body ample time to absorb and utilize the hormone.

Since melatonin supplements can help reset the body's internal clock, they can particularly be useful for people with jet lag or shift work related sleep disturbance. Nonetheless, they may not work for everybody, and if you're interested in trying them, you still want to make sure you're following good sleep hygiene practices, and not solely depending on their effects.

While melatonin is generally considered very safe, some people can experience some side effects such as nausea, lightheadedness, headaches, and dizziness.

5-HTP

5-Hydroxytryptophan, or 5-HTP for short, is an amino acid naturally produced by the body that functions as a precursor to Serotonin. Serotonin, a neurotransmitter, and the target of many anti-depression and anti-anxiety drugs, plays a key role in the regulation of mood and sleep. 5-HTP is a popular supplement used for its potential ability to promote relaxation, improve mood, sooth the mind, and enhance sleep quality. 5-HTP is available over the counter in many forms, such as pills, capsules, and liquid, and is generally a safe supplement for most people when taken in the appropriate recommended doses. However, high levels of serotonin can cause side effects like nausea, vomiting and diarrhea. For most adults, the typical dose will fall somewhere between 50 and 300 mg and should be taken in the evening before bedtime with a glass of water. Start with a lower dose and titrate up as needed.

Note that 5-HTP can interact with certain medications that affect serotonin levels and lead to dangerous ramifications. These include medications like some antidepressants and anti-anxiety pills, and so it's very important to speak with your doctor first and get their recommendations before starting this supplement, especially if you are on any medication or if you suffer from medical conditions like depression or anxiety that are related to serotonin levels.

While you do want to be cautious with it, 5-HTP in the appropriate dosing is still very safe for most people and can be of great benefit to many who are looking for supplements to help them sleep better and more effectively.

Magnesium

Magnesium plays a key role in many functions of our body, from the function of our muscular and nervous system, to blood sugar control, and blood pressure regulation. Importantly, magnesium also has a soothing and a calming effect on our nervous system. Therefore, it's a popular supplement for promoting sleep and relaxation. Studies show that a deficiency in magnesium levels is associated with sleep disruptions and lower quality sleep. Studies also show that magnesium supplementation may help enhance the quality and duration of sleep. You can find magnesium supplements over the counter in most health stores, and it comes in many forms such as magnesium citrate, magnesium glycinate, magnesium oxide, magnesium malate and others.

Magnesium citrate and magnesium glycinate are commonly available and are generally absorbed well and used to ease tension and promote relaxation. Magnesium oxide is a less costly type of magnesium, but the body absorbs it less efficiently.

Be aware that magnesium supplements might induce adverse effects such as diarrhea and nausea in some people, especially if used in excess. The recommended daily dose of magnesium for adults is between 320 and 420 mg; however, the optimum dose may vary based on age, gender, and overall health.

GABA

GABA (gamma-aminobutyric acid) is an amino acid that functions as an inhibitory neurotransmitter inside the brain. Low levels of GABA are associated with anxiety and sleep difficulties. Supplementation with GABA can be helpful in promoting relaxation, reducing anxiety and improving sleep quality and duration in some individuals. GABA is readily available in tablets, capsules, and powders. GABA dosing does vary widely depending on the product and the individual needs, so make sure you read the manufacturer's recommendations and check the label for directions.

In addition to supplementations, foods that are naturally rich in GABA may help increase its levels thus promoting relaxation and good sleep. Foods high in GABA include vegetables like spinach, cabbage and broccoli, bananas, berries, lentils, and fermented foods like yogurt and kimchi.

L-Theanine

L-Theanine is another amino acid that is commonly used as a dietary supplement to induce relaxation and relieve stress and anxiety with its soothing effects on the mind. It is a natural substance found in tea leaves and some mushrooms. According to research, L-theanine may also be good for enhancing sleep quality and reducing the time it takes one to fall asleep. It may also help mitigate some of the negative effects coffee can have on sleep. It works by increasing alpha waves in the brain, which are generally connected to a state of relaxation, and decreasing beta brain waves, which are associated with a state of alertness and activity.

Typically, the recommended dose of L-theanine is between 200 and 400 mg taken in the evening about 30 minutes before sleep.

Glycine

Glycine is a natural amino acid found in many vegetables, seeds, nuts, and meats. It functions as an inhibitory neurotransmitter in the brain and has been shown to have calming and soothing effects on the nervous system. Research has suggested that taking glycine supplements before bed can have positive effects on the sleep quality and shorten the time it takes one to fall asleep. It's also believed that glycine can help control the body's temperature during sleep, which is why supplementation may help reduce nighttime awakenings in some individuals. Glycine is generally tolerated well at appropriate dosages in most people with minimal side effects.

Tryptophan

Tryptophan is another naturally occurring amino acid, and it play a significant role in the production of serotonin. It's a precursor to 5-HTP, the supplement discussed above, and therefore can have some of the same benefits as it works through the same pathway. 5-HTP maybe more effective than tryptophan at increasing serotonin levels, but for those who can't tolerate 5-HTP tryptophan may be an option. As is the case with 5-HTP, you want to check with your physician before starting tryptophan especially if you're taking any other medications since tryptophan can a interact with certain medications, especially those related to serotonin levels and production in the body.

Inositol

Inositol is a naturally occurring carbohydrate found in many foods, and it plays an important role in many of our bodies' functions, including mood regulation and neurotransmitter signaling. Inositol can have calming effects on the body promoting relaxation and reducing tension, which in turn may translate into better sleep quality. While more research is still needed on the effects of inositol, studies suggest that, like 5-HTP and tryptophan, it may help control serotonin levels in the brain, which can also influence sleep. Foods high in inositol include whole grain bread, almonds, walnuts, beans, and peas.

B6 (Pyridoxine)

Vitamin B6, or pyridoxine, is a water-soluble vitamin found in food such as fish, poultry, chickpeas, and bananas. It plays an important role in the production and regulation of serotonin and melatonin levels. Research suggest that vitamin B6 supplementation can help enhance the quality and duration of sleep in some people. Vitamin B6 supplements are readily available and can be taken as capsules or pills. Keep in mind that too much B6, especially for prolonged periods of time, can have side effects so it's important to read the manufacturer's recommendations, and to take correctly and in the appropriate recommended dosages.

Zinc

Zinc is an essential mineral for many body functions, including immunological function, wound healing, and DNA synthesis. It also plays a role in sleep regulation. According to studies, zinc deficiency is associated with poor sleep quality, and zinc supplementation may enhance sleep quality and duration. In addition to playing a role in the conversion of tryptophan to serotonin, zinc supplementation may also lower the levels of cortisol, a stress hormone that can disrupt sleep. Zinc, at the appropriate dosages is generally safe, but excessive zinc consumption can have negative side effects, therefore it's important to take correctly and to always read the label on the zinc supplement products.

CoQ10

CoQ10, also known as ubiquinone, is an important and powerful antioxidant found in most cells of the body. CoQ10 plays an important role in cellular energy production and in cell and tissue protection. Studies show that the levels of CoQ10 go down with age and with other factors. Lower levels of CoQ10 are associated with multiple health issues including heart disease and diabetes. Some studies also suggest that CoQ10 supplementation may have multiple benefits on the heart, blood pressure and immune system among others. In some people CoQ10 may also play a beneficial role in improving sleep quality. CoQ10 is generally safe at appropriate dosage. While it can have many benefits, more studies on its effects on sleep are still needed. It can be worth a try because many people do report that it does help them sleep better. However, there are some people that report they prefer to take CoQ10 in the morning because it wakes them up and it can actually make it more difficult for them to sleep if taken too late. With this supplement especially, if you want to try it as a sleep aid, it's important to monitor how you're responding to it and adjust accordingly as everybody's reaction might be a little different.

Tart Cherry Juice

Tart Cherry juice, which is made from Montmorency cherries, also known as sour cherries, contains melatonin and is often used to help improve sleep. Research suggests that drinking tart cherry juice in the evening can enhance melatonin levels, resulting in increased sleep quality and duration. Tart cherry juice is also likely to have many additional benefits as it is rich in antioxidants and may help lower levels of inflammations in the body and improve general wellbeing. Keep in mind however, that tart cherry juice can be high in sugar, so make sure you choose a brand that does not include added sugars, and consume it in moderation.

While the supplement discussed above are generally considered very safe for most people in the appropriate dosing, they can cause side effects in some, especially if taken in excessive amounts or in susceptible individuals. Some supplements may interact with certain medications like benzodiazepines and SSRIs. Therefore, it's important to always consult with your healthcare provider first before starting any new supplements, especially if you're taking any other medications, are pregnant or breastfeeding, or have any medical conditions or concerns. Also keep in mind that the supplement industry is not as regulated as much as the pharmaceutical industry so the quality of the products can vary.

Therefore, make sure you're choosing high quality supplements from reputable sources.

The addition of supplements to one's evening routine can provide many benefits but should be done to complement one's healthy habits and sleep hygiene, not to replace them. It's not uncommon for people to start using supplements to help them sleep and then as their other sleep habits improve and their sleep routine gets more refined, they find that they don't need the supplement as much anymore to get a good night's rest. At that point they can either stop the supplement or continue it if they find it is also bringing other benefits since many of these supplements do have other health benefits outside of helping one fall asleep faster and longer as we've discussed. By selecting the appropriate supplements, and following good sleep hygiene, you can increase the quality and duration of your sleep and awaken feeling more rejuvenated. Keep in mind that the quality and safety of dietary supplements can vary greatly; thus, it is vital to do your research and select high-quality products from trusted brands that adhere to good manufacturing practices and third-party testing.

Chapter 11

Sleep Hacks for Better Sleep

While lifestyle modifications should be the cornerstone of good sleeping habits, there are several other quick hacks and techniques that can assist you in falling asleep faster and for longer. This chapter is dedicated to some of these tools and ideas including some relaxation techniques, breathing exercises, and tools like sleep masks and noise machines that one can you use to help them sleep better. These methods can be particularly useful for anybody looking for some quick results or who wants an extra boost on top of their other efforts. If you're looking for something you can start using tonight, this section is for you.

With the hectic nature of today's world, and the increased levels of stress and anxiety we often experience, getting a good night's sleep has become a more difficult task for so many of us. We've already discussed in the previous chapters ways to help deal with that stress and ways in which mindful meditation, yoga, and stretching can help quiet the mind and relax the body. We'll start this chapter by talking about a few other relaxation methods and techniques that you can use tonight to help you sleep better. The first one I want to briefly mention is progressive muscle relaxation which we've discussed in some details in Chapter 5. It can be a very useful approach to help one sleep better and you can use it tonight. This technique entails progressively contracting and relaxing different muscle groups in your body, beginning with your toes and progressing to your head. By doing so, you can release physical tension and produce a sensation of relaxation throughout your entire body, making it easier to fall asleep. There are a few other relaxation techniques that many people find useful, and we will discuss some of them below:

Autogenic Training

Autogenic training is a relaxation method developed in the early 20th century by the German psychiatrist Johannes Schultz. It utilizes autosuggestion to induce a state of calmness and to help alleviate tension and anxiety. Autogenic training is founded on the premise that the body has a natural ability to relax and repair itself, which may be accessed via concentrated attention and positive imagery.

Autogenic training entails assuming a comfortable position, sitting or lying down, and repeating a sequence of sentences or mental images to oneself. These sentences are meant to generate feelings of warmth, heaviness, and relaxation in different regions of the body, such as the arms, legs, and abdomen. The repeated use of these mantras and images can help develop a profound sensation of relaxation and calmness over time.

To try autogenic training for better sleep, find a peaceful and a quiet location. Close your eyes and take a comfortable seat or position on the ground, chair, or bed. Take several deep breaths to relax your body and mind. Next, concentrate on your body and the sensations you are experiencing physically. Repeat to yourself, beginning with your feet, a phrase such as "My feet are warm and heavy." Repeat this statement several times to yourself while visualizing warmth and heaviness spreading into your feet. Go on to the next portion of your body, such as your lower legs and calves, and repeat the process with a new sentence.

The goal is to create a feeling of warmth, heaviness, and relaxation throughout your entire body by focusing on one part at a time. After your calves, bring your focus to your thighs, then your glutes and so on, all the way to top of your head. As you progress through each body component, focus on deep, steady breaths and muscular relaxation. Try to let go of any distracting thoughts or concerns as you practice and allow yourself to totally relax into the process.

By the end of this practice, you should feel peaceful and relaxed. With repeated practice, autogenic training can be a powerful technique for enhancing sleep and general health. Therefore, it can be a helpful technique to start tonight and incorporate as needed into your nighttime ritual, letting your body and mind relax and prepare for a healthy sleep.

Guided imagery

Guided imagery is a relaxing method involving the use of one's imagination to create pleasant mental scenarios. This can help relieve tension and anxiety, making it easier for you to fall asleep. To try this method, find a quiet and comfortable area where you can lie down or sit comfortably. Close your eyes and start by take a few deep breaths to calm your body. Visualize a peaceful scene, such as a relaxing beach, a tranquil forest, or a calm lake. Envision the details of the scene and bring your attention to the sounds, sights, and smells in as much detail as you comfortably can. You want to envision yourself there, at ease, feeling peaceful, relaxed, and content. If you need help with this visualization method, there are guided imagery recordings you can find online that can help with the process. Some people also find it useful to repeat positive phrases to themselves like "I feel at peace and relaxed", or "I am filled with calm and tranquility". By focusing on these positive pictures and affirmations, you can move your attention away from racing thoughts and anxieties and into a state that is calmer and more relaxing. With practice, guided imagery can become a potent technique for inducing relaxation and improved sleep.

Relaxation techniques like autogenic training and guided imagery can be highly effective. These practices reduce tension and worry and soothe the mind and body, making it easier to fall asleep and remain asleep throughout the night. Some people may prefer the progressive muscle relaxation method or breathing exercises and find those tactics to be more useful. Choose the relaxation technique that works best for you taking into consideration your personal characteristics and preference. Try different approaches to find the one that helps you attain the most peaceful and refreshing sleep you can get.

Breathing Exercises

Breathing exercises can be another option for those looking for a simple and effective approach to help relax the mind and body. These exercises can help you fall asleep faster and experience a more comfortable night's sleep. In this section, we will examine three of the most popular breathing techniques that can be used for relaxation and sleep enhancement: 4-7-8 breathing, alternating nostril breathing and diaphragmatic breathing.

4-7-8 Breathing

4-7-8 breathing entails inhaling deeply for a count of 4, holding your breath for a count of 7, and exhaling gently for a count of 8. This approach can assist in slowing down the heart rate and inducing a sense of calm.

To practice 4-7-8 breathing, sit or lie down in a quiet and comfortable location. Take several deep breaths in order to calm your body. Next, inhale for four seconds through your nose, filling your lungs with air. Hold your breath for seven seconds, and then exhale through your mouth for eight seconds, so that your lungs are fully empty. This cycle should be repeated three more times, for a total of four breaths. Whenever you feel worried or nervous during the day, you may utilize 4-7-8 breathing to help relax your mind and body. The practice can be done with your eyes open or closed, but if you want to fall asleep faster at night, you may want to try it with your eyes closed. Some individuals find it beneficial to mentally count while performing this method in order to keep the correct tempo. If it is challenging for you to hold your breath for seven seconds, begin with a shorter length, such as three or four seconds, and gradually increase it as tolerated.

Alternating Nostril Breathing

Alternating nostril breathing, also known as Nadi Shodhana Pranayama, is a common yoga and meditation breathing technique.

This technique consists of inhaling through one nostril while blocking the other with a finger, then exhaling through the opposite side. This exercise is meant to help regulate and balance the body's energy by alternating the passage of air between each nostril.

To practice alternate nostril breathing, sit in a comfortable posture with your eyes closed and your spine in a neutral position. Use the thumb of your right hand to obstruct your right nostril, and inhale deeply through your left nostril for four counts. Hold your breath for four counts, then block your left nostril with your ring finger as you release your thumb and exhale through your right nostril for eight counts. Inhale for four counts via your right nostril, hold for four counts, and then switch back to blocking your right nostril while exhaling through your left nostril for eight counts. This sequence can be repeated for several minutes.

It is thought that alternate nostril breathing has a relaxing and balancing impact on the neurological system, hence reducing tension and anxiety. By focusing on your breath and the sensation of air passing through your nostrils, you can shift your attention away from racing thoughts and anxieties, thus encouraging relaxation and improved sleep.

Diaphragmatic Breathing

Diaphragmatic breathing, also known as belly breathing or deep breathing, is a relaxation method that reduces tension, promotes relaxation, and makes it easier to fall asleep. In contrast to shallow chest breathing, which utilizes only the upper chest, diaphragmatic breathing entails using the diaphragm muscle located below the lungs to breathe deeply and completely.

Choose a quiet area to lie down or sit comfortably to practice diaphragmatic breathing. Place one of your hands on your chest and put the other one on your abdomen. Take a slow, deep inhale through your nose, filling and expanding your abdomen like a balloon. Feel your abdomen and lower hand lift while your upper chest remains motionless as you inhale. Hold your breath for a few seconds, then gently exhale through your mouth, allowing your belly and hand to return to their original position.

Focus on your breathing and the sensation of your abdomen rising and falling for several minutes. Some individuals find it beneficial to counting their breaths as they go.

Diaphragmatic breathing can help relieve stress and promote relaxation throughout the body, making it easier to fall asleep. It can also be done at any time of day to decrease tension and promote tranquility and relaxation. With practice, diaphragmatic breathing can become a natural and effective go-to method for whenever you feel anxious and want to calm down your mind or fall asleep quicker.

These breathing exercises may be performed at any time and in any location, and they can be particularly beneficial when you are feeling nervous, agitated, or are having too many racing thoughts. By implementing these strategies into your everyday routine, you can learn to manage your breathing, lower your stress levels, and improve your sleep.

Visualization Techniques

Visualization techniques are powerful tools that can help promote relaxation and a more restful night's sleep. By creating relaxing mental images using your imagination, you can reduce tension and anxiety and prepare your mind and body for a pleasant night's sleep. We've previously discussed a potent visualization approach when we discussed guided imagery earlier in this chapter, but there are many other variants on this theme. Any form of visualization that helps you relax and calm your mind's racing thoughts down is beneficial. There are plenty of ideas and techniques you may come across online or through reading, but one particular visualization technique that is a classic when it comes to helping one sleep is counting sheep.

COUNTING SHEEP

The "counting sheep" approach is a well-known visualization method that has been used for a very long time to help people fall asleep. While its precise beginnings are uncertain, the method can be dated back to the Medieval Ages. This approach entails visualizing a relaxing scenario in which sheep are jumping over a fence one by one. While it may seem like a funny notion, the counting sheep technique can actually be quite useful, and it has been used for centuries to help individuals relax and go to sleep indicating that it can be a valuable and effective tool.

You can use this method when you're in lying in bed ready to go to sleep. Close your eyes and take a few deep breaths to help calm your body. Envision a green field with a fence. Imagine that there are white fluffy sheep in the grassy field. Gently and rhythmically, count the sheep one by one, as they jump over the fence. As you count, try to let go of any stressors and distractors, and keep your focus and attention entirely on the counting and on the visualization. If you mind begins to wonder, gently bring your attention back to the image and resume the counting. There are many variations of this method that have evolved over the years, from modifying the counting to other animals or objects, such as stars or clouds, to the addition of a peaceful mantra or phrase, like "I'm fully at peace", to the practice.

The counting sheep method is so effective partly because it works as a form of mental distraction. By staying focused on the work at hand, your mind is less likely to get caught up in racing thoughts and anxieties, which can keep you awake at night.

Ultimately, while the counting sheep approach may not be effective for everyone, it is a basic and easy-to-use visualization strategy that has stood the test of time and helped many individuals go asleep more quickly and receive the rest they need.

Sleep-Inducing Foods and Drinks

As previously noted in chapter 4, what you eat and drink can have a big effect on the quality of your sleep. We've already discussed that you may want to avoid having a large dinner or spicy food immediately before bed for example. Personally, I prefer not to consume any significant amount of calories within three hours of bedtime. I typically have a glass of herbal tea during this time since it can help me relax. A glass of chamomile tea or one of the other herbal teas we've discussed would be my typical drink of choice. There are always evenings, though, when late-night hunger strikes, and I feel compelled to grab a snack. Knowing that certain foods and beverages contain properties that might encourage relaxation and make falling asleep simpler makes my choices easier. In this part, we will examine some of these foods and beverages. While I still wouldn't advocate eating a large dinner too close to bedtime, if you feel the urge to eat or have a snack, you may want to consider one of the following:

Warm Milk is one of the most popular and classic sleep-inducing beverages. Milk contains tryptophan, an amino acid that plays an important and key role in the production of serotonin and melatonin; both of which are important for mood regulation and circadian rhythm balance. Warm milk before bedtime can help you fall asleep more quickly and enhance the quality of your sleep. However, for people who are sensitive to milk and dairy, such as those with lactose intolerance, this may not be the best option, and an alternative such as almond milk or soy milk, may be a better option.

Bananas are an excellent source of magnesium and potassium, two minerals that promote relaxation and can help alleviate muscle tension. A banana eaten before bed can aid in muscular relaxation and make it easier to fall asleep.

Almonds are abundant in magnesium which helps promote relaxation and reduces anxiety. A handful of almonds before bed may help relax the mind making it easier to wind down for bed.

Oatmeal is an excellent source of complex carbohydrates, and contain calcium, magnesium, and potassium. It can help stimulate the synthesis of serotonin and melatonin, thus a cup of oatmeal before bed may help promote calmness and sleepiness.

Cherries are a natural source of the sleep-regulating hormone melatonin. Before bed, consuming tart cherry juice or dried tart cherries may increase sleep quality and duration.

Walnuts are an excellent source of the amino acid tryptophan, which plays a key role in the production of serotonin and melatonin. A handful of walnuts consumed before bedtime may enhance sleep quality.

Kiwis are another natural source of many vitamins and antioxidants, and research suggests that consuming one or two kiwis about an hour before bed may help improve sleep quality and duration.

Turkey is rich in the amino acid tryptophan as well, and it is a good source of protein, which may also help contribute to good quality sleep. A small amount of turkey before bedtime may aid in falling asleep faster.

Sweet Potatoes are rich in potassium, which can help relax muscles and encourage sleep. In addition, they include complex carbs, which might improve your body's serotonin synthesis.

Like with anything else, it is essential to realize that not all foods and beverages are going to have the same effects on everyone. As previously mentioned, a cup of warm milk may assist one individual enjoy a better night's sleep, but it may have the opposite impact for those with lactose intolerance or dairy sensitivity. It is essential to pay attention to your body and experiment with various options to determine what works best for you. Tracking your response with a sleep diary is not mandatory, but it can be useful for documenting and monitoring which foods work better for you.

Tools for Better Sleep

The following are a few more tools and products that may help you fall asleep more quickly and remain asleep throughout the night.

SLEEP LIKE A BABY

Sleep Masks

Sleep masks are an efficient and simple tool that can help one in falling and staying asleep. A sleep mask is a soft, lightweight mask that covers the eyes during sleep, filtering out light to help create a dark, relaxing environment. Those who find it difficult to fall asleep in highly lit situations or those who are sensitive to light in general might benefit greatly from sleep masks. They are particularly beneficial for people who work night shifts or have an irregular sleep schedule, as they can simulate darkness throughout the day.

There are a variety of materials and styles for sleep masks, including silk, cotton, and foam. Some masks contain adjustable straps to allow for a comfortable and snug fit, while others may incorporate aromatherapy smells or cooling gel inserts. When you purchase a sleep mask, make sure you choose one that is comfortable, fits you well, and made of breathable material that won't excessively trap heat and cause sweating. When you use the sleep mask, make sure it is covering your eyes completely and not letting light in, while at the same time, it's not too tight. Adjust the straps if needed to get a comfortable fit. If it's too tight or uncomfortable, it probably won't be too relaxing and may interfere with your sleep instead of promoting it.

Because they're inexpensive and simple to use, sleep masks can be a great tool, especially for those who are sensitive to light or have to sleep in a lit environment. Sometimes it can take some getting used to for some people to get comfortable with wearing a sleep mask, but with time it can become an easy and integral part of ones' sleeping regimen. Some will find that the sleep can be very helpful when used with some of the other methods discussed here, such as guided imagery and certain breathing techniques.

White Noise Machines

White noise machines are designed to conceal ambient noise by emitting low-level, continuous sounds similar to a fan or a steady hum. The sound produced by a white noise machine is meant to mask other sounds like traffic and external noise that can disrupt your sleep. Those machines come in different shapes, size and forms, and with different sound producing abilities. You can find them online and at many electronic stores. Some will only emit white noise while others will give you many sounds to choose from including nature sounds or pink noise (which is slightly different than white noise but aims to have a similar effect of blocking other disturbing sounds). These machines can also vary in price, with some as low as ten dollars, and others costing several hundreds.

Using a white noise machine is usually easy and straightforward. Set it in the location you want and turn it on. Pick the sound and set the volume to the appropriate level if it's adjustable and let the machine do its thing.

A benefit of using a white noise machine is that it can help produce a more consistent sleep environment. In contrast to other noises in the surroundings, which may fluctuate and be unpredictable, the sound generated by a white noise machine remains consistent, promoting a sensation of tranquility and relaxation. Whether you live in a loud neighborhood or have a spouse who snores, the white noise machine can assist in creating a more pleasant sleeping environment. Additionally, some individuals find the sound of the white noise machine to be soothing on its own, allowing them to fall asleep faster and remain asleep for longer durations.

Look for a white noise machine that generates high-quality sound devoid of distortion and buzzing. You want to choose a machine that allows you to adjust the volume, and ideally gives you a variety of options in terms of the sounds produced, so that you try different settings and find the sound that works best for you.

Earplugs

Just like with sleeping masks, earplugs are a simple easy to use and affordable tool that can be used to help you block undesirable noises and fall asleep faster. These can be especially helpful if you live in a noisy environment, are a light sleeping, or are sleeping during the day. There are a variety of options when it comes to earplugs, from ones made of foam, to silicone, or wax, among others. The foam earplugs are the most popular and are made to be soft and spongy in a way that allows them to expand in your ear canal and block out external sounds. Silicone earplugs are typically more expensive but reusable and usually sit more externally blocking the entrance of the ear canal. Wax earplugs are also reusable and consist of a moldable, soft wax substance.

Consider the amount of noise reduction you require, as well as the fit and comfort, while selecting earplugs to purchase. Choose ones that feel soft and that are developed particularly for sleeping. You also want to make sure you're choosing a pair that fits snugly in your ear canals without causing irritation or discomfort.

Earplugs can be a useful aid for falling asleep and staying asleep, especially if you live in a noisy environment and don't have access to, or don't want to use, a white noise machine. Still, they're not optimal for everyone, and if you suffer from ear issues, are prone to ear infections, or to earwax buildup, then make sure you'd check with your doctor first before using them.

Body Pillows, Cooling Pillows, and Mattress Toppers

Body pillows are long comfortable pillows that are meant to provide extra support to the body. They can vary in style and shape, ranging from narrow to wide, and from straight to curved and contoured, but they are generally longer than ordinary pillows. They can be utilized to support a variety of postures to help increase comfort and enhance the quality of sleep. Some people find it restful to sleep while hugging the pillow, while others use it to support their legs or back. Certain body pillows are developed with pregnant women in mind and are meant to help ease pain and give additional support for the expanding belly.

Cooling pillows can assist in regulating body temperature and fostering a more pleasant sleeping environment. Sleeping in a warm or hot environment can make it difficult for some individuals to fall asleep and remain asleep. These pillows are meant to help draw the heat away from your body keeping you cool and comfortable. They are often made from permeable fabrics, such as cotton or bamboo, and frequently include a cooling gel or other heat-dissipating components. Some cooling pillows include changeable inserts that allow you to tailor the intensity of cooling to your preferences.

Mattress toppers, also known as mattress pads, are meant to add another layer of support on top of your mattress A comfortable mattress is necessary for a good night's sleep, but even the priciest mattress may not always deliver the ideal degree of comfort. Mattress toppers can assist in addressing this issue. These are thin, cushioned layers that lie atop your mattress to offer additional cushioning and support. Mattress toppers may be made from memory foam, latex, down feathers, or other materials. Some will also incorporate cooling technologies within them to help better regulate body temperature, prevent overheating, and keep a more cool and relaxed sleeping environment.

Sleep Tracking Devices and Apps

With the advancement of wearable technology, sleep tracking devices are becoming more and more popular. They can come in the form of wearable devices such as wristbands, smartwatches and rings, or as a standalone device that can be placed on the nightstand or under the mattress. There are also a variety of apps that can be downloaded to your smartphone that function to track your sleep as well. These devices and apps work by collecting and organizing data while you sleep, such as information about the duration and quality of your sleep, the time, spent in different phases of the sleep cycle, your heart rate, body temperature, breathing pattern, and/or the number of awakenings you experienced throughout the night. This way, they can provide valuable information that can be used to help you make adjustments and track your progress. Phone applications often make use of the accelerometer in a smartphone or tablet to track a person's nighttime movements and may utilize the microphone to detect snoring and other sounds that may disrupt sleep. In addition to recording sleep patterns, several sleep tracking devices and applications also provide tools to enhance sleep quality. Some devices may provide individualized sleep suggestions based on an individual's sleep data, while others may provide guided meditation or relaxation practices to assist users in falling asleep faster.

By providing useful data and giving personalized recommendations, these tracking devices and apps can be a beneficial tool for those seeking to enhance their sleep quality. Nonetheless, you don't want to solely depend on them, and you still have to take action and follow good sleep hygiene and some of the other advice provided here. And while sleep tracking devices and apps can be useful to some, they're not a mandatory constituent of a good sleep routine and like almost any technology, they have their downsides. Some may find them valuable, some may not. But it's a good idea to be aware of their availability, so that you can decide for yourself if they're worth a try. If you're interested, you can find these tracking devices online or in electronic stores. I will include some links in the resources webpage to some tracking device that will be regularly updated, as this is a continually evolving field, with new applications and gadgets entering the market and others leaving on a regular basis; therefore, presenting a list of specific apps here may not be especially useful, as the list may be out of date by the time you read this.

Getting Lots of Sunshine During the Day

Last but not least for this chapter, a key tool for achieving a better night's rest occurs throughout the day. We've previously discussed the significance of the circadian rhythm, your body's internal clock that tells you when it's time to sleep and when it's time to wake up, but we've mostly discussed it with reference to nighttime.

Nevertheless, if you're having difficulties sleeping, you may not have considered as a key factor, the amount of sunshine you're receiving during the day. Sunlight exposure throughout the day can help maintain our circadian rhythm regulated and in sync and increase the quality of our sleep at night. Moreover, getting enough sunlight throughout the day may improve mood, cognitive function, and general wellbeing. Sadly, many individuals do not receive sufficient exposure to natural light owing to a number of factors, such as working indoors all day, residing in places with minimal sunlight, or spending the majority of their time in artificial light.

If you're having trouble sleeping, it's crucial that you obtain enough natural light during the day. It is also crucial to note that even on overcast days, being outside and exposed to natural light can be beneficial. Here are some ways for getting lots of sunshine during the day:

1. Take a stroll outdoors during your lunch break.

2. Open your shades or curtains and sit near a window while you work if possible.

3. Consider investing in a light therapy lamp that resembles natural sunshine if you work from home or spend significant time inside.

4. Engage in some outdoor activities or hobbies that you find enjoyable (such as gardening, hiking, biking, playing tennis, golfing, etc.)

SLEEP LIKE A BABY

While getting enough sunlight is important and has tons of benefits, you still want to make sure that you are protecting yourself from the negative effects of UV radiation. Make sure you're using a sunscreen to protect all exposed areas of your skin when outside in the day, especially if you're out there for an extended period of time.

If you need help choosing the right pillows, sleep tracking devices, mattress pads and other tools we've discussed in this chapter, you can check out HealthMasteryLab.com/Sleep for more information.

Chapter 12

Other Notes & Special Considerations

No book about sleep will be complete without talking about napping. Sleep doesn't exclusively happen at night. Outside of napping, there are a couple of situations that often come up that are worth nothing; how to deal with jet lag and how to deal with night shift work. Both of these situations can have a significant impact on one's sleep and are worth diving into in some details. Finally, the use of a sleep diary has been mentioned already a few times in this book, but we haven't yet discussed this topic in sufficient details. This chapter will further explore these topics, starting with one that's not only common among humans, but among many animals as well, including cats, dogs, and dolphins, the act of napping.

Napping

Napping is a popular habit practiced by many people all over the world. Despite the fact that some people may see napping as a sign of sluggishness, research has shown that having a little nap can really be good for productivity and general health, since it can help reduce fatigue and enhance cognitive performance throughout the day. The timing and duration of the nap, however, does a play a role in its impact on sleep and general well-being. The optimum time to nap for most people is probably in the early afternoon, somewhere between 1 and 3 pm. This is due to the fact that your body naturally experiences a drop in energy levels around this time, which can make it easier to fall asleep and get the most of your nap. Napping much later in the day, particularly in the evening can actually negatively affect your ability to sleep later at night. Therefore, if you need to nap closer to your bedtime, try to limit your nap to no more than 30 minutes in length and try to keep it at least 4 hours from your bedtime. Keep in mind that the best time to nap will vary from person to person and will heavily depend on one's work and sleep schedule. For instance, somebody who works a night shift and usually sleeps during the day may find that the optimal time for them to take a nap is late in the evening or in the very early morning. The mid-afternoon nap tends to work best for people who follow more of a 9-5 schedule and go to sleep around 10 pm at night for instance.

Just like the best time to nap can vary, the ideal duration of each nap can also vary from person to person, and can be influenced by factors like age, lifestyle, and general sleep habits. That being said, experts generally recommend keeping most naps around 20-30 minutes long to allow enough time for the napper to feel a bit more refreshed and rejuvenated without going into deep sleep. This may be preferable over a 40 to 70 minutes nap for example, because with that slightly longer duration, you're giving your brain enough time to go into slow-wave, stage 3 deep sleep, but not enough time to complete a whole sleep cycle, which might cause you to wake up feeling groggy due to sleep inertia. If you have more time and want to nap more than 30 minutes, you may want to take an extended nap that lasts about 90 minutes. You can finish a whole sleep cycle in this amount of time, which can allow you to wake up feeling more refreshed. Yet as already indicated, if taken too late in the day, extended naps can also interfere with evening sleep.

As always, you want to pay attention to your body. Despite the fact that these basic suggestions are useful and will offer you a place to start, the best time to nap may simply be when you feel the most tired or worn out. The length of your nap will also vary depending on your preference and personal needs. To determine what works best for you, experiment with various sleep durations and periods while paying attention to your body's cues.

Having the ideal atmosphere for a nap can help you make the most of your nap, just as establishing a sleep-conductive environment can help you sleep better at night. You want a find a comfortable surface to nap on, whether it's a bed or a comfy sofa, ideally in a relaxed environment without too much noise, and at a comfortable temperature. Avoid napping in awkward uncomfortable positions or on the floor or other hard surfaces. Many people find that the use of a blanket during a nap can be helpful and comfortable. Some prefer silence while others like to have some soothing music or some white noise in the background. Try to limit external disruptions and distractions by turning off your phone or placing it on silent mode and use any of the previously discussed tools and methods as needed, such as progressive muscle relaxation, essential oils, a sleep mask, guided imagery, to help you relax and fall asleep faster. Finally, keep in mind that taking a nap does not replace getting a proper night's sleep. It can be a useful technique to supplement it, but it shouldn't be used as an excuse for poor or inadequate nighttime sleep.

Managing Jet Lag

Jet lag is a common problem that one might experience after a long flight due to the disruption in their circadian rhythm as they go across multiple time zones. As you traverse those time zones, your biological clock goes out of sync from the local time, and all the sudden it's still daytime when your body thinks it should be dark at night or vice versa. This can result in a number of symptoms like exhaustion, irritation, trouble focusing, and irregular sleep patterns. This disruption in your biological clock and sleep pattern can make it challenging to enjoy the trip or to quickly readjust to your regular routine. Fortunately, there are a few strategies you can apply to help minimize some of those negative effects.

While the main reason behind jet lag is the body's failure to rapidly adjust to the new time zone, causing a mismatch between your internal clock and the external world, other factors can also play a role. Dehydration, low oxygen levels, and travel-related stress are all elements that can worsen the body's disturbances, making it more challenging to overcome jet lag.

Here are some suggestions to lessen the effects of jet lag and help you make your travel experience more enjoyable:

1. Change your sleep schedule: Starting to alter your sleep schedule before your vacation might be useful if you're going across several time zones. Adjust your sleep time gradually toward the destination's time zone. Your body will be better prepared to adjust to the time change when you arrive if you do this.

2. Stay hydrated. Dehydration is a problem on its own, and it can make the symptoms of jet lag more pronounced, so make sure you

drink enough water when you're traveling. Avoid excessive alcohol and coffee since they can dehydrate you.

3. Use daylight to your advantage: Try to go outside and be in the sun during the day to receive some natural light exposure, which may help reset your body's circadian cycles. Avoid strong light in the evening if you're moving westward and try to get as much exposure to bright light as you can in the morning if you're traveling eastward.

4. Consider supplements: Supplements like melatonin and others we've spoken about can help in regulating your sleep-wake cycle. Refer back to that chapter if necessary and consider using a sleep-supporting supplement before bedtime in the new time zone to help you adjust quicker.

5. Avoid heavy meals and alcohol: These might reduce the quality of your sleep and make your jet lag symptoms worse. Try to avoid alcohol, and consume light and healthy meals when flying.

6. If possible, relax the first day: When you get to your destination, try to take it easy the first day and not to engage in activities that are too demanding. Before jumping into strenuous endeavors, give yourself some time to rest and to get used to the new time zone.

7. Have a regular sleep schedule: Once at your destination, try to stick to a regular schedule right away. This may help your body adjust more quickly to the new change.

8. Optimize your flight plan. If at all feasible, book a flight that lands at your destination in the evening time. Getting there in the evening, especially if you are a bit tired from the flight, will make it easier for you to go to bed right away. This will allow you to wake up feeling more refreshed the next day, with your internal clock already starting to adjust to the new time zone.

9. Change your sleep routine: As soon as you reach your location, make every effort to swiftly change your sleep schedule to the local time. Try to remain awake till bedtime if you arrive in the morning. Try to relax and go sleep at a good time if you arrive in the evening.

Overcoming jet lag can be a bit of a process, and it will come easier to some versus others. Some will adjust fairly quickly, while others may have to be a bit more patient as it can take a few days for their bodies to adapt and attune to the new time zone. But, with the correct strategies, you can help reduce these symptoms and prepare yourself more effectively for the time change.

Night Shift and Sleep

Shift work is a common phenomenon and it can have some advantages like higher compensation or greater flexibility, however, it can also have some negative effects on sleep and health.

Working night shifts may be difficult since it frequently requires turning your routine on its head and against your natural circadian rhythm, attempting to strike a balance between work and life when your body is urging you to sleep. This may result in restless nights, exhaustion, and other negative health effects.

There are however, methods that night shift employees can employ to help deal with some of these difficulties and enhance their sleep. These methods can lessen some of the detrimental effects of shift work on their health so that they can continue to have a fruitful and satisfying work life balance. By making a few changes to your routine and surroundings, like the ones listed below, you'd be able to enhance your sleep quality and general well-being:

1. Stick to a consistent sleep schedule: Strive to maintain a regular sleep schedule even on your days off. Your circadian clock will be better controlled as a result, and the quality of your sleep might improve. Try to get the 7-9 hours of sleep you need throughout the day to make up for the missed sleep at night.

2. Establish a sleep-friendly environment: Make sure your bedroom is dark, quiet, and cold. To reduce light, think about utilizing eye masks or blackout curtains. To block out any outside noise, use earplugs or a white noise machine.

3. Avoid Caffeine and stimulants: Steer clear of coffee and other stimulants in the hours leading up to your bedtime since they can make it difficult for you to fall asleep.

4. Use light to your advantage: Bright light exposure at the appropriate time can aid in regulating your circadian rhythm and

increasing alertness. Use bright lighting at work and make an effort to get outside during daylight hours if not close to your sleep time. In the same sense, use eye masks or blackout curtains to block out light when it's time to go to bed.

5. Take naps if necessary: A little nap might help you feel more awake if you're feeling sleepy or fatigued throughout your shift. To prevent them from interfering with your ability to sleep, keep naps brief (less than 30 minutes) and try to take them early in your shift.

6. Consider melatonin and other supplements: Melatonin plays a major role in regulating your sleep-wake cycle. Using melatonin or a similar supplement before your scheduled sleep time, along with the other methods discussed here, might help you wind down and make it easier to fall asleep.

7. Stay hydrated: Make sure you drink enough water throughout your shift. Fatigue, weakness, difficulties in concentration, headaches, and other health issues can all worsen with dehydration.

8. Exercise: Doing regular exercise will help you sleep better and feel better overall. Vigorous Exercise shouldn't be done too close to bedtime though because it might make it difficult to fall asleep. Any form of exercise done in proximity to your sleeping time should be gentle and relaxing.

9. Eat a balanced diet: Good nutrition is crucial for maintaining your general wellbeing and energy levels. Consume a balanced diet that is high in fresh vegetable, healthy fruits, lean protein, and whole

grains. Avoid eating large meals or spicy food right before bed since they might make it harder to fall asleep.

10. Avoid smoking and alcohol: Smoking and excessive alcohol usage can harm your general health and your ability to restfully sleep. If you're a smoker, think about quitting, and if you're drinker, keep it in moderation.

11. Use relaxation and stress management techniques: Night shift work can be demanding and stressful for the mind and the body. Refer to chapter 5 for ideas that can help you manage your stress levels and promote calmness and tranquility. Use these methods and techniques as needed to help you relax and sleep better.

12. Consider a light therapy lamp: For some people who work night shifts, light therapy might be a valuable tool to regulate and enhance their sleep. The goal of light therapy is to mimic the natural cycles of light and dark that our bodies are accustomed to. During the work shift, using a light box that emits strong light can help balance the body's circadian cycle and encourage alertness. For the same reason, you'd want to avoid exposure to bright light before you want to go to sleep, whether that is in the morning or afternoon for you. It can also be a good idea, if you're using light therapy at night, to progressively cut back on light exposure as the night shift progresses towards its end, to signal to the body that it's time to wind down and get ready for bed. If you're buying a light therapy lamp,

make sure to select one that can emit the appropriate amount of brightness and that is designed for night shift usage.

Using these methods, you can lessen the negative effects of shift work and schedule changes on your sleep and general health. Your body may need some time to get used to different schedules, but with persistence, patience, and the appropriate routines, you can get the deep sleep you need. Adjusting your sleep schedule and getting used to the night shift can come easier to some versus others, but with a little patience and some trial and error, you can find the approach that works best for you. It's also always a good idea to express your concerns to your employer and look into any reasonable accommodations that can help you cope with shift work better.

Sleep Diaries

An efficient strategy to monitor your sleep habits and spot any problems that could be impairing the quality of your sleep is to keep a sleep diary. A sleep diary is a daily journal in which you keep track of your sleeping patterns, lifestyle choices, and daytime moods and activities. It can help you spot where improvements may be needed and how your sleep habits are affecting your overall health.

You can use a physical notebook, a digital notebook or spreadsheet, an app, or wearable technology as a sleep diary. Since I don't like to use any digital screens or applications right before bed and right when I wake up, which are two times you'd want to record in your diary, I personally prefer the more traditional method of keeping a physical diary and a pen.

You should record the time you go to sleep and the time you wake up each day. Include all naps you take and write how long each one lasted. You'd also want to record the number and duration of any nighttime awakenings you experience. In addition to those details, you should also keep track of other elements that could affect the quality of your sleep. These include lifestyle choices and routines such as your food intake, especially close to bedtime, your exercise regimen, coffee and alcohol consumption, as well as other tools we've covered in this book, such as documenting any relaxation techniques, supplements, or essential oils that were used. By keeping track of these elements, you may start to see patterns and connections emerge between your lifestyle choices and your sleep quality, and the effects and patterns of your sleep habits may become better understood. As you start to implement new techniques, habits, and lifestyle modifications, this process will also help you track these changes and see if they're working for you of if you need to make further adjustments.

A sleep diary can be a useful tool for anyone who wants to take that extra step to help optimize their sleep and monitor their habits and progress. You can either create your own diary at home or buy one online. You can find a printable log and some recommended links and tools at the book's resources webpage on HealthMasteryLab.com/Sleep. Monitoring your sleep, tracking your behaviors and improving your routines can not only help your sleep, but it can help improve your overall health and wellbeing as well.

Chapter 13

Conclusion

Getting a good night rest is not only crucial in order to feel rejuvenated and revived throughout the day, but it's also a cornerstone of good health. Sleep is an integral part of living a healthy life and is essential for preserving our physical and mental well-being, so it should be given the attention it deserves. It also allows us to perform at our best throughout the day. For maximum efficiency and productivity, our bodies need time to rest, heal, and revitalize. Sadly, problems with sleep, including insomnia, are all too frequent. Without enough sleep, it's likely that we'll end up feeling tired, unable to concentrate, and even our immune system can be weakened. Luckily, there are several tools and methods one may employ to improve their sleep: whether it's improving their sleep environment, keeping a regular sleep routine, adding relaxation techniques, or incorporating natural remedies and sleep promoting hacks. By adopting some of these tools and techniques, you can develop a healthier sleep habit that works for you and allows you to get the deep rejuvenating sleep you need.

In order to build your optimal sleep routine, it's helpful to start by evaluating your existing sleep habits and patterns. This will assist you in identifying areas for development and in establishing realistic goals. Take a step back and evaluate your existing habits objectively. Look at the whole picture and take into account things such as your diet, the amount of alcohol or caffeine you consume and their timing, your exercise routine if any, the amount of sunlight you get each day, the quality of your sleep environment and so on.

Start by asking yourself questions like:

• What time do I generally go to sleep and what time do I wake up?

• Is it difficult for me to fall or remain asleep?

• On average, how much sleep do I get?

• When I wake up, do I feel refreshed and rejuvenated or drowsy and worn out?

• Are there things such as noise, light, or distractions, that prevent me from sleeping well?

• What is the quality of my sleeping environment? (Is the room cool, quiet, and dark? Do I have soft and comfortable pillows and mattress? Etc...

- When is my last meal usually, and what is my regular diet?
- Do I adhere to my sleep routine consistently?
- Do I have a relaxation routine that helps me get ready for bed? Does it work for me?
- Do I receive enough daylight during the day?
- How much caffeine do I typically get and how long before bedtime?
- How much alcohol do I typically drink and how long before bedtime?
- Am I spending too much time on screens and getting too much blue light before bed?
- Etc...

By answering these and similar questions, you can get a deeper understanding of your present sleeping habits allowing you to better pinpoint areas that need improvement. For instance, if you frequently have trouble falling asleep due to stress and anxiety at bedtime, it can be worthwhile trying some of the relaxation techniques previously discussed. Or you may discover that the days when you have caffeine past a certain time are the days where you can't sleep well and suffer from more nighttime awakenings. You may start to see certain relationships between activities you do throughout the day, like shows you watch or foods you eat, and the hours of sleep you end up getting that night. Although it is not essential for success, maintaining a sleep diary even for just a week or two may be a very useful tool to assess your current habits and patterns.

After evaluating your present sleeping patterns and identifying areas of improvement, the next step to take your sleep to the next level is to create clear, attainable goals. Your goals need to be practical and catered to your unique situation and needs.

Prioritize the changes that you think would improve your sleep the most. For instance, buying earplugs or a white noise machine may have a greater effect than altering your night routine when external noise is the major issue. Conversely, if you have trouble relaxing before bed or falling asleep at night due to racing thoughts, then implementing relaxation techniques may be your main approach.

Keep in mind that although certain changes can be simple and easy, others may need more time and work. Buying and adding a supplement before bed can be quick and simple, but some lifestyle modifications, such as reducing your coffee intake or modifying your diet, can take much longer to complete. For these bigger goals, starting with smaller, more manageable objectives and working your way up gradually to more major changes can be a great approach. For instance, if you often drink a lot of coffee in the evening, a manageable objective may be to convert to decaf or to cut back by one cup a day. Setting a time frame, whether it be a week, a month, or more, for completing some of these more challenging lifestyle goals is also beneficial. This can keep you inspired and allow you to monitor your development over time. Be kind to yourself and remember that progress might not come right away.

While everyone might take a slightly different approach, it's typically a good idea to take both types of changes into account when it comes to sleep improvement. Look for techniques and methods that are quick to put into practice that can be started right away, such as purchasing blackout curtains, maintaining a cool bedroom temperature, buying a particular essential oil, consuming one of the herbal teas previously mentioned, or incorporating stretching, mindful meditation, progressive muscle relaxation, or one of the other quick relaxation techniques we've mentioned in the book. At the same time, you should also be honest with yourself about some of the other lifestyle choices we've discussed, decide which ones are worth improving, and create a strategy and a schedule for changing those bigger and more difficult goals as well. As you proceed, keep an eye on your progress and adjust as needed. By evaluating your present sleeping habits, defining goals and priorities, incorporating natural remedies and hacks, and tracking your progress, you can significantly enhance not only the quality of your sleep by your health and well-being overall.

Always remember that getting enough good quality sleep is not only important for your overall productivity, energy, and happiness, but it is essential for your physical and mental health as well.

Prioritize your sleep and establish a relaxing sleep environment and you'll start to see the benefits to your health and well-being.

Take advantage of this book's advice, prioritize your sleep, and live a life filled with more rest, peace, health, and energy.

Sweet dreams!

This Page Intentionally Left Blank

Download your free companion guide including a sleep log and find additional resources at HealthMasteryLab.com/Sleep

About the Author

Family doctor and anti-aging expert Dr. Adam Well has helped people of all ages adopt a healthier lifestyle, fight symptoms of aging, get relief from common ailments, and live healthier happier lives. Outside of seeing patients in his clinics, Dr Well enjoys sharing his knowledge through the seminars and workshops he provides for other physicians and healthcare providers from all over the world. He is all too familiar with the toll that sleeplessness can have on a person's wellbeing and daily functioning. Dr Well's fascination with sleep disorders began when his mother suffered from insomnia. He was determined to help her and studied sleep science extensively, and his own bout with the disorder strengthened his resolve to assist others in overcoming their own sleep issues. In his book "Sleep Like a Baby," He shares his wealth of knowledge and expertise in the field, in the hopes of enhancing the readers' quality of sleep through a simple and natural approach.
For more information visit
Www.DrAdamWell.Com

www.ingramcontent.com/pod-product-compliance
Lightning Source LLC
Chambersburg PA
CBHW020425220526
45464CB00002B/571